Health, Ethnicity and Diabetes

Harshad Keval

Health, Ethnicity and Diabetes

Racialised Constructions of 'Risky' South Asian Bodies

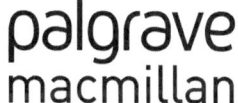

Harshad Keval
Canterbury Christ Church University
Canterbury, Kent, UK

ISBN 978-1-137-45702-8   ISBN 978-1-137-45703-5   (eBook)
DOI 10.1057/978-1-137-45703-5

Library of Congress Control Number: 2016938691

Cover image © Bobu Nicolai / Alamy Stock Photo

Printed on acid-free paper

This Palgrave Macmillan imprint is published by Springer Nature
The registered company is Macmillan Publishers Ltd. London

"For Asesha, Tayen and Ayana"

Acknowledgments

I would like to thank the following people for their support, encouragement, humour, intellectual interaction, and patience. The intellectual process of writing this book is really about the culmination and emotional processing of my history—one which has been shaped by wonderful, and sometimes adverse, circumstances. I would like to thank the following people who have played a part in shaping this journey: at Preston College, Martin Holborn, for never giving up on the 'real gone kids.' Katherine Tyler, Martin Bulmer, and Frank Pike at Surrey; My friends and colleagues at Canterbury—Daniel Smith, Julia Carter, and Matthew Ogilvie—for their support and friendship throughout the process, thanks. My thanks also go to Holly Tyler and Dominic Walker at Palgrave for their help and patience. Without the people in the communities on which this book is based, the study would not have taken place; so, my sincere thanks for the time you all took to be with me, and for your warmth. Finally, to my simply wonderful family—Asesha, Tayen, and Ayana—thank you for your patience, constant laughter, and smiles—the light in the darkness; and for being a constant reminder of all that ever is, and ever will be, important.

Contents

1

Introduction

This book is about the relationship between health, race, and ethnicity, and how people manage their experiences of type 2 diabetes, using a variety of tools located in their social and cultural contexts. More specifically, the book also aims to explore how the relationship between health and ethnicity in the UK has developed over the last few decades. These developments have witnessed a number of racialising tendencies, occurring at policy, political, and individual experiential levels. While the book is about the experience of diabetes amongst groups of South Asians in the UK, it is, more importantly, an analysis of the ways in which the health states of minority groups have become racialised in different ways and at different times. How people think about their health and illnesses, what they do about them, where they seek help—the array of impacts from socio-economic and structural factors and the long-term effects of these are all part of the rich intellectual and academic history of medical sociology and anthropology. In this book, I am focusing on how a condition such as diabetes becomes both part of everyday life for people, and also shows us how health and illness conditions are part of wider, socio-cultural processes. I often refer to these processes in this book as 'constructions of risky South Asian bodies'. By this, I mean that in parallel to

© The Editor(s) (if applicable) and The Author(s) 2016
H. Keval, *Health, Ethnicity and Diabetes*,
DOI 10.1057/978-1-137-45703-5_1

(not over and above) the daily experience of diabetes-related symptoms, seeking diagnosis and treatment, thinking about the impacts on one's life, and using one's cultural and ethnic identity to manage and deal with the illness are larger, overarching processes which shape people's experiences. I want to contextualise people's experiences within a socio-cultural framework that acknowledges that there are processes of discursive construction in operation. I define discursive practices as a series of actions that involve, over time and space, ways of thinking, conceptualising, viewing, writing, and impacting.

My mention above of 'risky South Asian bodies' is a term I use to signpost a series of discursive practices. There is a discernible pattern within health science discourse, which includes government policies and guidelines, academic literature within both biomedical and social sciences, as well as media representations, which have linked the racialised, ethnic, cultural, and social category of 'South Asian' to diabetes. There appears to be a widely accepted common-sensicality within academic public health discourses about the 'racial', 'ethnic', and/or 'cultural' nature of diabetes. Placed in the context of a number of wider issues, this emerges as a problematic relation for a number of reasons. *First*, there is an existing problematic relationship between Black and Minority Ethnic (BME) communities and health in the UK, which still in the process of being resolved. *Second*, as evidence over the last 40 years has established, general racial discrimination, differential access to healthcare, problematic attitudes to BME communities within healthcare services, and health promotion campaigns which have focused on specific 'cultural' traits of communities have all had a lasting impact on the health of BME groups in the UK. *Third*, there is a vast array of data, which indicates that on many socio-economic levels, BME communities suffer from structural, formal, and informal inequalities in opportunities in education, employment, housing, and healthcare. *Fourth*, the global and national burden of diabetes has rapidly increased at what most government agencies, media outlets, and academic writers regard as an alarming rate. This worldwide increase in diabetes becomes the backdrop health panic to more national and localised sets of panics. However, these health panics, of which diabetes is but one (obesity is another separate, but intimately related, health scare), are also characterised by ethnic and cultural specificity. In other words, although there is a *generality* to diabetes panics, that is, 'the whole world is at risk', the power and influence of expert knowledge systems, such as epidemiology, have proved beyond any 'rational' doubt that *some* groups are more at risk than others. In this book, I do not intend to debate the epidemiological evidence, although this is the subject of contestation. Rather, I examine what has been written about South Asian groups and diabetes, and what the symbolic and practical significance of this might be. The data generated as part of this study then shows us how we can locate people's experiences in relation to discursive constructions. Talking with individuals, groups, observing people in situ, generated data which not only demonstrates what and how people do for the everyday management of diabetes but also gives us an indication that what some agencies call 'culture', or 'ethnicity'—deemed fixed possessions that give apparently straightforward information to observers and researchers—are actually far more complex. They are what Neal et al. (2013) see as living multiculture, and subject to flex and change as the complex layers of socio-cultural and political interactions take place. In a sense, I am identifying how constructions of risky South Asian bodies are actively *resisted* in people's everyday lives. On one level, official discourse and health practice in a wide range of interfaces (GP surgeries, community health centres, hospitals, etc.) create, maintain, and perpetuate specific versions of what it might mean to be South Asian and have diabetes. Usually, this involves having a vague 'genetic' risk (even though there is no known specific genetic mechanism identified as yet), and also, in tandem, being 'culturally' at risk (the belief/understanding that some groups do not engage in exercise and good diets, in addition to their beliefs and non-compliance with biomedical regimes).

As people are given the opportunity to talk and reveal their thoughts, feelings, and practices, the often simplistic, reified, and static way in which race, ethnicity, and culture have been treated in the health science discourses is rendered as dynamic, malleable, and adaptive as people navigate their complex socio-cultural landscapes. Constructions of South Asian diabetes risk require specific elements in order for these representations to be effective in discourse. Within this book, I point towards a number of specific elements we can identify. Culture and lifestyle are popular mechanisms, and indeed, metonyms used by discursive agencies to both explain and prepare the ground for associated treatment. I take particular issue with the way in which BME groups become identified as 'culturally' deviant in both their health choices and the related lifestyles they are perceived to have. These simplistic categories of 'culture' and 'lifestyle' also include diet and exercise, as well as people's attitudes to using official biomedical forms of healthcare. Again, within this work, and as published elsewhere (Keval 2009a, 2015), I argue that, within the field of 'race' and health, the drive to establish causal explanations has often pathologised people's cultures. This form of 'cultural pathologising' (Ahmad 1996) renders cultural and ethnic identity—a dynamic processual feature of all human social formations—static, creating fixed identities generated through stereotypes, incorrect assumptions, and possible discriminatory attitudes. Groups defined as 'minorities' then become categorised as having certain cultural faults, which lend themselves to higher health risks. The follow-on impact of this in terms of health intervention is, of course, diagnosis, treatment, and in parallel, health promotion campaigns. The crucial element here is that if the underlying conceptualisation of ethnic and/or cultural identity is simplistic and often problematic, then all of these related entities will also be subject to this problematic underwriting—a racialised gaze. With a condition as widespread in discourse and in people's lives as diabetes, the importance of re-aligning this gaze becomes rather important.

A final element to the construction of South Asian risky bodies lies in the more recently ratified 'new genetics' arena. Diabetes, as Mcgee and Johnson (2013) point out, is not a single disease, but a cluster of conditions. While bio-scientists of many specialities have demonstrated their expert knowledge base in its mechanisms and associated disorders, there has yet to be a fundamental causal explanation for why some groups might be more susceptible than others. Genetic predisposition has long been a feature within the range of possibilities in high-risk BME group identification. Whilst early studies in Southall, London indicated six-fold increases in diabetes risk amongst South Asians (Mather 1985; Eapen et al. 2009; Barker et al. 1982), the causes of these increased risks could not be established. As I mentioned above, awareness of the condition, early detection, appropriate treatment, as well as dealing with perceived 'barriers' to healthcare, such as language, 'cultural' attitudes, and lifestyle factors such as lack of exercise and poor diets, were the main focus. However, in recent years, a parallel focus has emerged, and is gaining both widespread support and momentum—the genetic predisposition of South Asians to higher diabetes risk. Its importance is clear in the way in which South Asian diabetes has undergone a number of racialised and culturalised gazes, notwithstanding the great array of excellence in health intervention at all levels of healthcare. A new direction of diabetes risk has developed. My aim is to identify these discursive processes, and again, highlight the way the lived, experiential practice of social and cultural action provides people with the means to actively manage their conditions, but also, demonstrably *resist* the narrow confines of simplistic culturalised and geneticised pathology. I discuss some salient and emerging issues in the new genetic—racial diabetes discourse as they relate to the South Asian 'risk-package', and return to this in more detail in the Conclusion.

Within this study, a range of social, cultural, and biographically embedded diabetes stories emerged. The conceptualisation of the illness, the diagnostic process, the role of diet and nutrition, exercise and help seeking for the condition, and the role of biographies and histories in connection with community and place all became part of the stories and narratives that contextualised diabetes. These aspects, however, are not treated as isolated and static representatives of a medical model of disease management; rather, they are situated within the social and cultural contexts of lived social action. Allowing these stories to emerge provides a way to situate diabetes and the constellation of its impacts within a wider social and cultural landscape, and one which reminds us of the myriad ways in which people negotiate their lives. The picture rendered is not just a descriptive account of 'what people do'. Rather, what concerns this study is the role cultural, social, and ethnic identity plays in facilitating the management of and coping with the disease. Locating the work within this framework also involves the exploration of migration-related settlement experiences, biographies, and existing connections the group has with the countries or continents they lived in prior to migration (usually, Africa and India). The stories which emerged in participants' accounts framed the active construction of identity, rather than passive acceptance of identities, which have been maintained by caricature and reification of concepts of minority cultures and groups. A consistent theme I return to is the troubling and persistent relationship between health and race, as materially and discursively performed in a number of practices. The resultant manner in which health becomes 'racialised' through a re-codifying of 'cultural signifiers' is worthy of critical appraisal.

Throughout the book, I employ concepts of ethnicity, culture, and difference critically, so that the dynamic ways in which these ideas are used in people's everyday practices are reflected. These notions of 'difference' and 'sameness' form the backbone of the methodology, and employ as their core concept a system of identity dialectics. Accessing individuals and groups, places and spaces, required negotiations of the delicately balanced terrain of '"insider" outside' identities. Notions of identity within the research process are also subject to the ebb and flow of social action. These 'cultural validations' (Keval 2009a, b), a process of engagement and interaction of researcher and participant identities, allow for the interconnectivity of biographies and identities by making explicit the 'researcher-researched' relationship. There is an invocation here of the possibility of treading on the wrong side of identity absolutism—that is, you have to share absolute characteristics to carry out the research and generate these findings. However, this is neither the intention nor the stance taken here. The emphasis is on the role of cultural identity in research, and how various explicit connections between the researcher and the researched can, in the best traditions of general human relationships, enhance the research process. It is not by polarising the argument between value-free, culture blind approaches and supposed 'authenticity' that this debate can progress. Rather, unpacking the possible connectivities and what this may mean and come to symbolise for all parties is where some interesting insights might be gleaned.

While it is clear that in incidence and prevalence rates, to use the lexicon of epidemiology, there are clearly higher proportions of people categorised as South Asian with diabetes than White and other ethnic categories, it is problematic that neither 'culture' nor 'genetic predisposition' have been proven in any way to be part of the causal chain. And yet, the messages circulated by networks of health science discourse as well as popular health iconography (one only needs to look at posters for diabetes prevention, or websites providing information about high-risk groups) are that if a group's 'culture' is modified, and their 'genetic' makeup accepted, then all would be well. This book principally seeks to undermine this assumption and contest these discourses, which are, as Foucault summarised, 'practices that systematically form the objects of which they speak' (1972: 49).

Outline of the Book

This book is divided into two parts. The first introduces, then explores, the ways in which constructions of culturalised and racialised risk play a role in the ethno-diabetes arena. In order to do this, I discuss health policy and academic research to focus on how notions of culture, lifestyle, and genetic factors are seen to be playing a role in South Asian diabetes. Part 2 aims to show how participants in this qualitative study demonstrably activate counter-narratives to these discursive constructions through the use of a variety of different cultural and socially embedded tools in their repertoire.

Chapter 2 locates the study within the general concepts and ideas used in the discussion of health and ethnicity. Rather than explicating foundational concepts, I aim to contextualise the ways in which health, ethnicity, and South Asian identities may be usefully explored. This necessarily requires that we look at how race and health have been treated in the past within academic and non-academic discourses. Chapter 3 first situates the sociological exploration of diabetes as a contextual, nuanced, and complex physiological disorder, whose varied and multifactorial impacts on people's lives can only really be understood through the lenses provided by sociologies of chronic illness. It then goes on to provide a picture of diabetes in terms of prevalence and incidence. The expert knowledge base of epidemiology is a contestable issue; nevertheless, I maintain that we can use this knowledge base critically. By this, I mean that we can acknowledge the various processes of construction that go into the operationalisation of variables of ethnicity and race; as Montoya (2011) has boldly pointed out, the genetic and race diabetes industry is no stranger to this process. We still need to know, in the interests of appropriate health intervention (in the face of people suffering from the condition), crudely, the numbers involved. In other words, we must have a sense of how many people are suffering from the condition, and what, if any, might these 'singularising' characteristics be. Chapter 4 explores how through the use of various discursive techniques, a combination of lifestyle and genetic predisposition arguments have been mobilised to construct the South Asian diabetic risk. The chapter discusses a number of relevant areas— epidemiological, general health science-related, and sociological. The aim here is to frame the study so that, first, a 'construction' of South Asian risk can be discerned, and second, a critique can be applied to the health science discourse which has generated this construction. Chapter 5 is an account of the general qualitative methodology employed within the study, and discusses both the philosophy and mechanics of the approach and its utility in this case. In this chapter, I also frame some epistemological concerns within the contexts of difference, culture, ethnicity, and identity. The aim here is to examine some of the ways in which aspects of my identity—occupying researcher as well as other roles—interconnected with roles and identities held by participants, and the impact of this on the research. These 'cultural validations' were central to the work, connecting with current debates within anthropology and sociology.

As I mentioned above, diabetes is not a single disease, but a constellation of symptoms, events, and processes—biological and socio-cultural. Chapter 6 begins with this starting point of the initial diagnosis of diabetes and the resulting prescriptive normativity, which is then associated with this. In other words, once a diagnosis of diabetes is established, depending on the type and severity, of course (this book is principally about type 2 diabetes), people are required to manage the condition in specific ways, but also, manage exercise and diet routines. These are, in reality, significant features of everyday life with resulting barriers, obstacles, and successes, and social action-related formulas which people generate *within* their own lived experiences. My aim is to show that while health science discourse constructs a rendition of South Asian people as generally requiring focused education, guidance, and emphatic encouragement to exercise and regard 'their' diets as needing modification, participants in this study demonstrably resisted these constructions of non-compliance or 'cultural deviance'. They show that these mechanisms for management are already embedded in their everyday cultural accomplishments.

Chapter 7 then looks at what kinds of treatments people seek, but importantly, frames these within a context of biography, experience, and cultural adaptation. Within both traditional medical sociology and anthropology, one of the main concerns over the development of these subfields has been what people do while seeking help for a condition. 'Help seeking' behaviour (Zola 1973) is a general conceptual and theoretical term used widely in social anthropology of medicine, cultural epidemiology, and medical sociology, and is related to the concept of illness behaviour (Mechanic 1978). As people conceptualise, monitor, and adapt to their own bodies, their 'illness, as well as illness experience, is shaped by sociocultural and social-psychological factors, irrespective of their genetic, physiological or other biological bases' (Mechanic 1986: 1). The early days of medical sociology and 'race' emphasised quantitative evidence, for important empirical reasons. Now, in the early decades of the twenty-first century, qualitative medical sociology has, potentially, a conceptual and theoretical grounding for exploration of how ethnicity and 'race' also play crucial roles in help seeking, illness behaviour, and the dynamics of culture. The treatment or help that people seek is not usually confined to one type or sort, just as people's attitudes, beliefs, emotions, and social connections are usually more complex and multi-layered. South Asian groups bring, certainly in terms of migration histories, a range of different ideas and information sources, which they then utilise and call upon in a complimentary and negotiated fashion, rather than in an exclusionary and static manner.

Chapter 8, in a sense, aims to set the experiences of diabetes amongst South Asian groups within broader notions of identity, community, and belonging. As Ahmad (1996) has argued, the use of simplistic, static notions of 'culture' and 'ethnicity' in health strips away all the dynamic properties of social action. As the preceding chapters try to show, human social actors experiencing health and illness conditions are far from static epidemiological or genetic categories. Rather, as Stacey (1988) informs us, people 'draw on all sorts of knowledge and wisdom, some of it derived from their own experience, some of it handed on by word of mouth, other parts of it derived from highly trained practitioners' (Stacey 1988: 142), including ethnic and cultural identity. This chapter then contextualises the space and place involved in managing diabetes, locating the cultural, ethnic, and biographically symbolic, and practical dimensions involved. The way in which people talked about communities, biographies, and their personal and cultural histories represent the ways in which, despite the constructions of South Asian risk that have been built up over a long period of time, people 'resist' these discourses, and prove that they utilise the varied, social and cultural resources around them to accomplish social action. Chapter 9 performs somewhat of a misleading function at this point in the book's narrative arc, because it takes us back to some of the discursively constructed regimes of biological and scientific truth I touched upon in the early chapters in Part 1. Here, I provide some discussion on the role of genetics in redefining 'racial' and ethnic identity within the diabetes arena, especially as it applies to South Asians in the UK. A number of socio-political processes have underlined the ways in which these genetic 'truth' making practices have gained momentum and legitimacy. I contest the absolute nature of these truths—nuanced and considered discussions in the field notwithstanding—and detail the pitfalls of this recoding of biological and cultural markers of difference. In Chap. 10, I provide some concluding comments.

References

Ahmad, W. I. U. (1996). The trouble with culture. In D. Kelleher & S. Hillier (Eds.), *Researching cultural differences in health* (pp. 190–219). London: Routledge.

Barker, D., Gardner, M., & Power, C. (1982). Incidence of diabetes amongst people aged 18-50 years in nine British towns: A collaborative study. *Diabetologia, 22*, 421–425.

Eapen, D., Kalra, G., Merchant, N., Arora, A., & Khan, B. (2009). Metabolic syndrome and cardiovascular disease in South Asians. *Vascular Health Risk Management, 5*, 731–743.

Foucault, M. (1972). *Archaeology of knowledge*. London: Routledge.

Mather, H. M. (1985). The Southall diabetes survey: Prevalence of known diabetes in Asians and Europeans. *British Medical Journal, 291*, 1081–1084.

McGee, P., & Johnson, M. (2013). Diabetes: A public health issue for the twenty-first century. *Diversity and Equality in Health and Care, 10*, 135–138.

Mechanic, D. (1978). *Medical sociology.* New York: Free Press.

Mechanic, D. (1986). Editorial: 'The concept of illness behaviour: Culture, situation and personal predisposition'. *Psychological Medicine, 16,* 1–7.

Montoya, M. J. (2011). *Making the Mexican diabetic: Race, science, and the genetics of inequality.* London: University of California Press.

Stacey, M. (1988). *Sociology of health and healing.* London: Routledge.

Zola, I. (1973). Pathways to the doctor: From person to patient. *Social Science & Medicine, 7,* 677–678.

Part I

Contextualising the 'Risky' South Asian Diabetic Body

2

Conceptualising Race, Ethnicity, and Health

In this chapter, I would like to explore some concepts that will be relevant in our discussion of health, ethnicity, and diabetes. Diabetes is, first and foremost, in the lives of individuals and groups, a concrete, tangible, and embodied entity. This means that, as social scientists, we cannot avoid the very real impact it has on people's lives, nor can we avoid the aggregate picture of incidence and prevalence. With the number of people with diabetes growing globally, exploration of social epidemiology becomes an integral part of the picture. Sociologically, I am interested not just in how we can use these empirical entities but also in how we can observe the discourses within which they sit.

Before moving to the relationship between South Asian people and the diabetes discourse, it is necessary to contextualise this within the overall discursive arena where it is located. Both the epidemiological and experiential aspects of health and illness are a feature of the landscape of racialised health, and so, I will start by looking at concepts and approaches in the health and ethnicity areas. This necessarily brings into focus a historical gaze, as multicultural health concerns automatically require the presence of multiple cultures within a given polity. For writers such as Bhopal, 'the key to understanding ethnicity and race in multi-ethnic societies is

© The Editor(s) (if applicable) and The Author(s) 2016
H. Keval, *Health, Ethnicity and Diabetes*,
DOI 10.1057/978-1-137-45703-5_2

immigration' (2006: 500). The nature of the health–ethnicity discourse, therefore, is a dynamic and politicised one, experienced by people in relation to their cultural, ethnic, and material positioning. I do not intend to repeat or rehearse the now considerable literature on multiculture, ethnicity, diversity, and health in the UK; these can be found elsewhere (e.g. Ahmad 1993; Bhopal 2007; Smaje 1995, 1996; Bradby 2003, 2012; Bloch et al. 2013). However, it is necessary to formulate health–ethnicity understandings against the backdrop of how a nation deals with 'difference'. With this in mind, I will explore a number of pertinent issues in race and ethnic relations in the UK before attending to how categories of difference in health might be thought through.

Conceptualising Race and Ethnicity in Health

The links between race, racism, and health are analysed and explored in sufficient detail in many excellent sources; however, it is relevant to briefly outline some of the main issues here for reasons related to the recirculation of what Paul Taylor called 'race thinking' (Taylor 2013). There are enduring legacies in the connection between biological, essential based 'race', on the one hand, and 'culture' and ethnicity, on the other. 'Cultural difference'—or 'diversity' as it is often labelled—is a multifaceted and polysemantic term, since it is used interchangeably with race, ethnicity, culture, and BME communities. It has, in many ways, become a metonym, and in Hall's powerful use of racialised signs analysis, a contemporary 'floating signifier' (Hall 1996). The shifting semantic grounding for the language of difference has played a substantial role in health and race. Whilst the traditional connections between race, science, and biology do not appear in as overt a form as they have in the past, the notion of 'culture' seems to have fitted neatly into the empty signifying placeholder. An ill-defined set of ascribed characteristics becomes the content of the 'culture difference' container and, as Ahmad and Bradby tell us, becomes referred to as 'primordial, innate and immutable' (2007: 797). Culture regarded and used as a new version of 'old' race thinking is not new, and is what Barker (1981) called the 'new racism'. Contemporary discussions of the complex relationship between health, ethnicity, diabetes, and South Asians, therefore, are contextualised by this conceptual and theoretical ground.

The crucial element to providing a nuanced discussion of culture, ethnicity, and health is to avoid regarding these ideas as fixed and unmoving, but rather regard them as dynamic and expressive of self-identity as 'boundaries of inclusion and exclusion between groups are negotiated...' (Chattoo and Atkin 2012: 23). As I try to link these notions to health, diabetes, and South Asian populations, it has become ever more important to note these fluidities within social interactions as self-identity (cultural, ethnic, or otherwise) mediated by power relations and struggles over resources (Hall 1996).

'Bio-race Thinking'

Any discussion of culture and ethnicity necessarily needs to be prefaced by and embedded within the wider ideas and practices of 'biological race thinking'. The invocation of blood or genealogical connection has been a fascination for many different biological, historical, political, and social sciences. Bio-race and health have a long and troubled history, and as the nineteenth century progressed, the measuring of bodies of people deemed to be of a lower civilisational order was a scientifically justified tautology (Malik 1996). The civilising and capitalist machinery which then forged the British and European colonial empires relied on this biological, intellectual, moral, and religious 'fixing' of 'races'. As Bauman (1989) has written in his sociological critique of modernity, the instrumental rationality involved in modernity made the scientific justification of attributing differential values to human lives possible. The resulting Jewish Holocaust (and other atrocities across the globe) was, therefore, in the logic of social engineering in Nazi Germany, both reasonable and desirable (Bauman 1989). The perversion of Darwin's original framework of evolutionary science led to social Darwinism, and the establishment of various Eugenics movements (Clarke 2006). The connection between eugenics, race, and society are by now clear—in Bauman's language, the 'gardening state' (1989: 20) is one where a particular vision or societal order is invoked, designed and planned for optimum order, delimited by entities that belong, and entities that do not. In this manner, political and emotive notions of nation, fatherland, racial purity, and *volksgemeinschaft* (Clarke 2006) bonded with the fullest maturity of technology and bureaucratic processes, resulting in systematic mass extermination. A second example I want to use to show how notions of bio-race can be implemented systematically, and with full official governmental approval, is the infamous Tuskegee Syphilis Experiment. Between 1932 and 1972, over 400 Black African American men were the subject of an experiment conducted by the United States Public Health Service. These subjects were not informed they had the disease, nor given any information about the effects. Most importantly, while the pharmacological industry had established the efficacy of the only known drug cure—penicillin—the men were neither informed about the same nor given any treatment. As Jones (1992) reported, the study's purpose was to map the biological territory of the disease—that is, stand by and watch how the disease affected this group of Black men. There was, at the time, a great deal of fascination with African American sexual relations, and the rates at which infected people might have sexual relations with other infected people, so the ostensible 'scientific' aims of the study, purportedly steeped in medical ethics, were actually related to what Clarke (2006) would call a darker, psycho-social set of racialised processes.

The parallels to what Bauman above identified as systematic, bureaucratic, modern, techno-rational processes are clear—in this case, interlinked with American race relations and struggles for African American civil rights. These examples of science applied to the study of human biological mechanisms used racial difference as a way not only to describe categories of people, but to explain their constructed inferiority and justify their objectification (Bhopal 2007). Race as a biological, fixed, immutable marker of difference was shown through a variety of European, Enlightenment-informed discourses to be scientific, rational, morally valuable, and most importantly, a 'fact'. When we are exploring contemporary treatments of racialised/culturalised discourses in South Asian diabetes risk construction, the conceptual machinery invoked has a historical, epistemological, and conceptual origin, steeped in centuries of 'othering' discourses. To try to discuss how 'cultural' and 'ethnic' differences might play out in contemporary arenas, we need this 'back story', because as the adage goes, the actors may have changed, but the play remains essentially the same.

Of course, gazing upon these ideas as the artefacts of knowledge and power production allows us to view any accepted knowledge as just one of a range of possible discursive outcomes. From a constructionist viewpoint, scientific objective truths *become* objective truths when treated as such by people who represent the interests of that approach. Race and health have an inheritance, which has been dogged by this coupling with racism, colonial power, and constructions of biological advantage. Certainly, as Lentin (2014) has shown, the fundamental philosophical and epistemological basis for newly emergent visions of 'European' rationality were deeply entrenched in raciological manifestations of othering. Ahmad and Bradby (2007) point out that the pseudo-scientific category of 'race' was sanctioned by science and religion (Christianity), which then led to the justification of oppression, such as slavery and bonded labour. Much of the justification was driven by the civilising missions of the Christian West, whose ostensible purpose was to bring morality and civility to 'heathen' and 'savage' pre-modern forms of life (but underwritten by the huge profit-generating strand of early capitalism). Western colonial oppression over the last four centuries has relied on the racialised literary, scientific, cultural, and political construction of 'other' peoples as essentially, biologically, intellectually, and morally inferior (Said 1977). The historical involvement of health within this programme of representation and practice is not incidental, but rather, instrumental. For example, during the Atlantic colonial slavery trade, *drapetomania* was an official diagnostic classification for the irrational desire of a slave to run away (Littlewood and Lipsedge 1989), and decolonisation was seen as ostensibly negative for 'races' of people who would not be able to adequately handle full independence (see Craig 2010 (in the bibliography) for concise summary).

While the current trend in South Asian diabetes discourse is to emphasise 'cultural' deficits and deviance (a point I develop later), there is still an influential legacy of race thinking in the 'new genetics' of diabetes (Keval 2015). I have included this section on the legacies of 'bio-race thinking' in order to contextualise the presence of both particular types of health thinking, and the presence of groups of people who were—and indeed, still are—the object of specific 'racial gazes'. A racial gaze objectifies the subject totally in terms of biological, essential, and fixed characteristics—ideas which have already been discussed above. This racial gaze, however, becomes transformed into 'cultural gaze', whereby the health deviance (e.g. non-compliance with 'good' health guidelines) is blamed on a 'faulty' culture. As I explain later in relation to diabetes and South Asian people in the UK, these forms of gaze are powerfully directed at people who have already had a history of racialised objectification. In Malik's (2009) summary, race, science, and medicine are intimately connected in ways which have endured well beyond what ethical considerations would require. Much of this legacy is alive and well in health service and policy (Bloch et al. 2013), and as I aim to show in this book, there are impacts on people's lives. As one of the components of scientific knowledge production, epidemiology has played a pivotal role in how racialised categories are used in research. Despite warnings from senior epidemiological figureheads, such as Bhopal (2006, 2007) and Krieger et al. (2005), research into links between health and ethnicity necessarily needs to tread carefully over conceptual, theoretical, and methodological terms, as much research is un-theorised (Nazroo 1997). In other words, research and intervention practice must take into consideration the complexities in labels that are used to classify people, the concepts of difference that are put into operation, and the links that might be made with health. Other writers have written about the power of epidemiology to strip away social, cultural, and political contingency from complex social entities, and leave reified results in their wake (Krieger 1994). Diddier Fassin eloquently summarises a range of complexities here: 'Ascription is the foundational act through which racialisation is produced. It is the imposition of difference.' (2011: 422) Such racial ascriptions are in parallel social, since recognition and misrecognition are mediated by relative social and economic positioning.

'Bio-moral Panics'

Alexander aptly argues there is no place for 'culturalist heat-and-serve' explanations (2004: 147). The racialisation of health has a duality to it: on the one hand, the marginalisation of BME communities at social and economic levels and the resulting marginalisation of needs; and on the other hand, the 'ethnicisation' (or over-culturising) of illness (Bloch et al. 2013). Most scholars in this area can agree that in the history of health and ethnicity in this country, there are a number of cases or specific campaigns which highlight the main issues I have outlined above. Ahmad (1993), Ahmad and Bradby (2007, 2008), and Bloch et al. (2013) have all pointed to a number of historical campaigns, which demonstrate examples of 'over culturalising' (Nazroo 1997) or cultural pathologising (Ahmad 1993). As Ahmad and Bradby (2007) summarise the fields of health and ethnicity by locating the notion of cultural pathology in two examples, here, I similarly use these two cases to illustrate my point. The first was related to the incidence of rickets in South Asian communities in the UK in 1970s (Rocheron 1988; Donovan 1984), while the second was connected to the issue of consanguinity (marriage between blood relatives) within Muslim communities (Ahmad et al. 2000). In both cases, the identified 'cultures' were culpable for living within practices deemed harmful to themselves, without any connection between them. In other words, the cultural sphere became the 'fault-sphere' of these groups, and in this way, the conditions underwent a process of racialisation. Rickets, a condition caused by Vitamin D deficiency, was already endemic in Britain in the middle of the twentieth century. Effective proposed solutions were outdoor facilities for children, vitamin-fortified margarine, and free milk. As the disease incidence increased in the recently arrived South Asian populations, it became 'exoticised' as a disease connected solely with minority cultures, through deficits in South Asian diets and dress codes. Other assumptions, as Ahmad and Bradby (2008) retell, were that dark skin was too pigmented to convert sunlight into Vitamin D. Rather surprisingly, the solution which was offered to White British children—fortified margarine—was never explicitly an option for South Asian children, regardless of its effectiveness. The only possible solution was the adoption of Western diets and lifestyles, both clearly the normative moral and cultural ideations against which 'foreign' cultures were set (Rocheron 1988).

The 'Asian Rickets' debacle was closely paralleled by the national 'biomoral panic' of intermarriage amongst blood relatives in the Muslim community. The urgency around this issue was triggered by high rates of infant mortality because of congenital problems in babies born to women of Pakistani origin. Despite the then growing evidence that much of the mortality should also have been viewed in light of material disadvantages, access to healthcare, age, migration—all factors which have been shown to have huge adverse effects on a wide number of health indicators (Nazroo 2003)—it was the single 'cultural' feature of intermarriage which was identified as the main reason. There is yet to be a unified, evidence-based causal link between consanguinity and infant congenital abnormality, yet there has been considerable interest, fascination, and attention from health and scientific communities, resulting in the stigmatisation of ethno-religious communities. As Ahmad et al. (2000) showed in their study, even without evidence of causal mechanisms, consanguinity has been showcased as 'explaining' a range of conditions in South Asian communities. I would contend that to this list of historical cases (for another example, in the case of sickle cell thalassemia, see Anionwu and Atkin 2001), we can conceivably add diabetes as another condition that has become an object of specific culturalising and racialising gaze through a variety of discursive practices.

Categories and Labels of Difference

In a comprehensive review of the relationship between health, 'race', and ethnicity, Smaje (1995) argues that in its unproblematic usage, 'race' is an 'ideological' category, imbued with socio-political and historical constructions. However, when 'race' is used as an 'analytical' category, it provides useful information about how people in various groups fare in terms of health status—including experiences of health and illness, and access to healthcare. As Sheldon and Parker (1992) observed, often, the mere description of ethnic differences evolves into an explanation of these differences, rooted in ethnic and cultural practices. One of the conclusions from many authors in this field, including Smaje (1995, 1996), Ahmad (1993), and Nazroo and Karlsen (2002), is that experiences of health and illness cannot be separated from the socio-political arena, and the combination of cultural and material environments people find themselves in. The simplistic use of culture and ethnicity as static and unchanging ideas has been vigorously critiqued (Ahmad 1993; Smaje 1995; Bhopal 1997). There is also the resultant loss of explanatory power in research, caused by rigid notions of what it means to belong to a specific cultural and/or ethnic group and the assumed related behavioural mechanisms involved (Kelleher 1996). There is a need to credit individuals and groups of people in society with agency, with the specific need in health and illness for elaborating how people demonstrate their agency, and its relationship with other social forces.

Studies which do not reify culture and ethnicity, but instead, 'reanimate' static ideas of identity are increasing, although the initial momentum which occurred during the 1990s in terms of empirical, analytical, and theoretical progress seems to have decreased. During the last couple of decades, commentators such as Ahmad (1993, 1996), Hall (1992), Stubbs (1993), Nazroo (1997), Nazroo and Karlsen (2002), Smaje (1995, 2000), Lambert and Sevak (1996), and Kelleher (1996) made significant contributions to the study of health and ethnicity, through empirical findings and their theoretical location. It is within the arena set by many of these renderings of the health and identity relationship that this study situates itself. As Nazroo et al. (2007) point out in their exploration of race, inequalities in health and differential experiences of material positioning, patterns, and contexts of migration are crucial. Treating ethnicity as an unproblematic, easily packaged variable in health analysis, where categories such as 'Caribbean', 'Black', and here, of course, 'South Asian' can be simplistically seen as representing some form of global universality, needs to be problematised.

'Culture' is often understood as a static entity—encompassing many different aspects of identity, including religion, faith, language, ethnicity, and class. The health professions in the UK, which intend to research communities where prevalence and burden may be high, but understanding still lacking, can assume that health behaviour and health status may be determined by something called 'culture'—as yet, unverifiable. As Lambert and Sevak argue, 'culture is made as much as given' (1996: 149), pointing to the conceptual fluidity which takes into consideration new circumstances, life events, observations, and information. The homogenised category of 'South Asian culture'—however it may be defined by 'external' sources—is often blamed or held partially responsible for illness and disease in these communities without substantial or theoretically robust evidence. The many conceptual, theoretical, and empirical advances in the study of race, ethnicity, and diasporic communities reveal anything but simplistic and mono-dimensional experiences (e.g. Ali et al. 2006; Brah 1996). As discussed earlier, South Asian 'culture' is far too quickly paraded as the responsible charge for many diseases and ailments (coronary heart disease, diabetes, rickets, and obesity). Indeed, as Lambert and Sevak (1996) note, in terms of vulnerability to cardiovascular disease (CVD), health messages, and behavioural change, there are striking similarities between White British and South Asian British people talking about their health experiences, leading one to conclude that the clumsy use of 'culture' to explain illness within a specific group simply is not robust enough. An important consideration which I have mentioned above, and the subject of much focus by Waqar Ahmad, is that of researching 'culture' and ethnicity in relation to specific diseases. Lambert and Sevak warn against: 'isolated observations...about particular health problems...Without reference to the broader, often non-health specific, cultural constructs, social determinants and individual histories in which...(lay) ideas are embedded...' (1996: 153). The need for approaches which account for socio-cultural and historical contexts to people's ideas about health and illness has become an urgent priority in medical sociology, but as commentators are keen to point out, sociology has arrived late to this arena (Ahmad 2007, 2008). In the next chapter, I explore specific knowledge bases relating to the diabetes experience to examine how these important socio-cultural backdrops to people's everyday life-contexts have been used.

Framing diabetes as a vehicle to explore how facets of people's cultural and ethnic identity are used to actively negotiate a landscape may fill in the gaps left by much previous research. Some of the more sophisticated studies have indicated that there is a universe of meaning to be examined in looking at the social and cultural experiences of illness (Kelleher 1996; Lambert and Sevak 1996). This context points towards there being an active and dynamic element in the resulting accounts people produce. This suggests that a different story about diabetes and South Asian people can emerge, perhaps as a counter-narrative, that does not negate the physiological impact or the plethora of excellence in research and intervention, but rather asks us to move beyond the limitations of unitary and static understandings of UK multicultural society. That story indicates that people, all human social groups, utilise their migration biographies, life experiences, and their 'designs for living' (Becker 1986) in ways which are socially and culturally fluid, but still retain powerful symbolic and practical markers of identities. Certainly, in this study, participants' notions of being Gujarati, Hindu, and British, their overseas connections, and their ways of finding remedies in different systems to deal and cope with their illness were part of these designs for living.

Ahmad warned against the tendency for the ideological basis of 'culture' to be used in a form which when 'stripped of its dynamic, economic, gender and historical context…becomes mechanistic, and determines people's lives—actions and behaviours, instead of being a flexible resource for living, according meaning to what one feels and experiences' (1996: 190). Using concepts of 'cultural difference' as a way of explaining facets of social experience—such as inequalities—effectively is a diversion away from structural inequalities and racism in peoples' lives. The focus on the entity called 'culture'—usually a loosely and/or ill-defined idea at best—employs taken-for-granted assumptions in research due to a racialised agenda. This is specially the case in the dominant epidemiological approaches that purport to be value-free and objective. As Ahmad points out, BME communities are expected to structure their needs to suit healthcare professionals—rather than the other way round. As Sheldon and Parker (1992) argue, healthcare professionals have a need to look at the way in which racialisation has determined the social, economic, and epidemiological location of people, a driving feature of much important recent work (e.g. Wohland et al. 2014; Bhopal 2013; Nazroo 2003).

Ethnicity then, for writers such as Kelleher (1996) who use a Weberian framework to situate this aspect of identity, is a structure of relevance used by people in a variety of ways in their everyday lives. By analysing this, it is possible to ascertain how differences between groups—the culturally different constituents of multiculturalism—have a role in how people manage their situations. For Kelleher, ethnicity is a non-essential and constructed entity, made as much by people themselves as others in the dynamics of power relations. In a similar viewpoint to Lambert and Sevak (1996), culture, for Kelleher, is a 'dynamic entity, which changes to incorporate fresh ideas and perspectives as people develop new ways to respond to their environment' (1996: 71). The way in which Kelleher draws upon sociological theory in order to explore identity through diabetes experiences is still relatively rare, although recent work examines this area and creates useful links with healthcare provision (Lawton et al. 2005; Greenhalgh 2005), and these do provide some interesting viewpoints regarding the experience of type 2 diabetes among South Asians. Lawton et al. (2005), for example, report how the use of oral hypoglycaemic agents (OHAs) among Pakistani and Indian participants was mediated by a trust in the efficacy of British medical systems. Knowledge and experience of remedies from the Indian subcontinent also influenced the decision—something which has resonance with this study. The findings strike a chord with this study since the decisions that people made were about negotiating the condition in terms of the particular context they found themselves in, which fluctuated, depending on their needs and perceptions. Some of these factors were, as Lawton et al. (2005) argue, 'cultural' as they were related to their ethnic identity, and influences attached to this—such as knowledge and experience of remedies from the Indian subcontinent. This, however, contrasts with Greenhalgh (2005), who, having also conducted extensive research into diabetes, mainly among the Bangladeshi population in London, argues that this should not be seen as primarily a 'cultural difference', but rather, as 'human nature', and suggests the patient's level of health literacy is more important than 'culture'. In terms of relevance for this study, this is important because the history of health and ethnicity research has demonstrated that often differences in health status between groups are explained by this poorly defined notion of 'culture' (Rocheron 1988; Dominelli 1988; Ahmad 1993).

While the application of labels of difference can be involved in unbalanced power relations, it is also possible to see this as a two-way process, as Nagel (1994) argues, who applies the symbolic interactionist approach to discuss the notion of 'symbolic ethnicity'. The view that groups will also have their own role in defining themselves in terms of ethnic and cultural identity is drawn upon in this study, since people's accounts of what they do with their diabetes, who they connect with, and how they see themselves in a social framework of living can tell us a great deal about how notions of identity are both stable and in flux. As Hall (1992) has argued, the idea of a single and fixed identity is a fantasy, which simply serves to comfort us in the postmodern era—the narrative of the 'self' is a construction of the period we live in.

The way in which difference is characterised, treated, and then used in research is, of course, principally an ontological question. That is, if the very conceptualisation of what difference means—for example, defining South Asian people's beliefs about diabetes and notions of inevitability—is categorised as a culturally fixed set of relations, then findings from research which uses these notions will most likely reveal fixed states of being and identity, no doubt suggesting that these 'cultural' findings point to a group of people being hindered by their 'culture'. Despite critiques, there is a persistent lingering of these static ideas. The ease with which fixed, rigid, and static characterisations of people are used acts as an incentive—a conceptual 'one-stop shop'.

Epidemiology and Ethnicity: A Numbers Game?

In 1993, Waqar Ahmad wrote in his introduction to *'Race' and Health in Contemporary Britain*:

> There are two main trends in research and writing on Black people's health. One is a vehemently 'culturalist' approach, where realities are constructed and explained in terms of cultural differences…The second approach is of supposedly benign epidemiology, the notion of an unconcerned, value-free scientific observer making objective pronouncements on the basis of carefully collected evidence which uses rigorous scientific methodology. (Ahmad 1993: 1)

In the twenty-first century, the arena of health and ethnicity has changed considerably, both in methodologies employed to collect/generate data, but also conceptually and ideologically. There now exists an extensive array of research at a national level in terms of policy, and also at localised levels. However, there is an enduring legacy of both cultural pathologisation—as Ahmad coined the phrase—and an epidemiological sense of infallibility (Krieger 1994). South Asian diabetes is both a medical certainty (an issue I explore later), explained, treated, and characterised in terms of biomedical concepts and also a cultural, social, and biographically located condition in the way that the concept 'culture' is used. As diabetes, obesity, and cardiovascular problems increase worldwide, a critical gaze in this arena becomes not just an interesting alternative to simple 'culture'-based and strict epidemiological models, but rather an essential component in nuanced understandings.

Epidemiological models offer statistics indicating rates of illness, while genetic theorists combine their arguments with 'culture' arguments in order to explain these rates of the illness. Since a substantial proportion of the research into health and ethnicity has been of the biomedical and epidemiological type, the focus has consequently been on populations and comparative analysis. The idea of relative risk, therefore, becomes a focal point around which much of the conceptualisation, data generation, and interpretations revolve. Conceptually and epistemologically, there are issues here, since comparisons in health issues are made using research-categorised minority groups, and a specific ethnic category of majority norms—usually called 'White'. This implies that minority health is only an issue in comparison to other groups, rather than as interesting and important in its own right (Ahmad and Bradby 2007). The idea of 'raised incidence or prevalence' in minority groups, regardless of whether or not this is an issue within the group itself, is an additional problem. The example Ahmad and Bradby use is tuberculosis, where rates remain high in some minority groups, but because of effective treatment, and importantly, the fact that overall, the prevalence rates are low, there is little attention paid to this. Cancer, however, provides a different set of challenges, since deaths from cancer represent one-sixth of all deaths in minority groups, and yet, this is paid little attention because, overall, the prevalence is lower than in the White population. The idea of relative risk rears its epistemologically challenging head here, and forces us to look at diabetes from a different perspective. While rates are clearly higher in the South Asian population, it is primarily this notion of 'relative risk' that appears to drive the over-whelming *bio-moral panic* amongst health science experts. The *heightened* risk amongst South Asians is, within the paradigm of epidemiological 'neutrality', an appropriate issue of concern, but given that diabetes also represents a worldwide burden of disease, there appears to be a duality in the working paradigm. On the one hand, everyone, globally is at risk of 'Western' lifestyles, but curiously, some are more at risk than others. Michael Montoya, in his ethnographic study of 'Mexican' diabetes, echoes this point. The focus of Montoya's work is partly his notion of 'bio-ethnic conscription', which, summarised, is the complex and subtle process of transforming ethnicity into something which is 'meaningful for scientific research' (2011: 158). Interestingly, in Montoya's study, it is explicitly not a study of diabetes as a medical condition, but as a study of the people who have come to be written into the racialised genetic discourse of diabetes, through the systematic meaning-making processes of science.

In this book, I am not only interested in how the participants in this study 'make meaning' within the everyday experience of diabetes as they negotiate multiple social, personal, and cultural landscapes. I am also concerned with how these active, dynamically charged agentive actions can be juxtaposed with health science's constructions of ethnic/cultural/racial/genetic/passivity and a sense of inherent weakness and deviance. There is meaning-making at both ends—for the subject and the discursive process of constructing the subject. Whilst I discuss the perpetuation and recycling of genetic arguments below and in Chap. 9, for Montoya, the 'circulation of racialised genetic material' (2011: 158) is key to how 'Mexican diabetes is made'. One of the keystones, however, to building the 'diabetes vulnerability' artifice is population studies, and as I discussed earlier, the notions of risk, prevalence, and incidence become quite central to the topic. There is little question that diabetes is an extremely complex disease, involving multiple causal and triggering factors. For Montoya, and the case of Mexican disease construction, there is a convoluted 'representational slippage' (2011: 159) demonstrated in the way in which US census data is *not combined* with epidemiological data to show 'relative risk'. In other words, US census data shows approximately 18 million White diabetics in existence, which, as Montoya points out, is four times the numbers for all African American diabetics, three times more that Hispanic rates, and 37 times more than American Indians and Alaskan Native diabetics. For the US context, there are 1.6 times as many White diabetics as all the groups listed above *combined*. And yet, diabetes is a powerfully racialised disease, constructions of which are legitimised by scientific models and authority. We can begin to discern how the socio-political underpinnings of health science discourse can steer both conceptualisation and practice in research and health intervention when race thinking is mobilised in specific ways.

The Bio-politics of Difference and Health

The wider political and ideological debates regarding 'difference', race, ethnicity, and culture are, of course, pertinent to this study, since the intention is to follow a narrative and social action thread from the individual's story of diabetes, through their connections with other people, places, and institutions. Weaved into this account is also the connection the person makes with accounts of their own history—migration and settlement, education, work, and positive and negative experiences in the UK—all acting as contexts and 'buffers' which mediate their health and illness states. 'Pathologising culture' rests on the shift from overt racism, based on blood purity and genetic types, to 'cultural' differences. The sense of essentialism remains the same, since minority groups are constructed as dangerous to themselves and can only be saved by becoming more like another group—perhaps the indigenous majority. The 'problematisation' of minority health leads discourse to generate solutions focused on binaried states of normal/pathological trajectories.

Compliance and deviance therefore in relation to prescribed modes of health behaviour become the all-encompassing solution base. BME communities are urged to attend to and follow the advice given by healthcare providers, whilst the providers themselves are armed with an array of 'cultural tools', which allegedly will bring about sensitivity (working on the assumption that a little sensitivity can solve problems of a deeper, wider ideological, socio-political, and economic nature). Such sensitivity has been the focus of interesting research, for example, Hilton et al.'s (2001) study on the traditional health practices of South Asian women in Canada, confirming that traditional practices were not used at the exclusion of medical remedies, and that health providers needed to be more culturally sensitive. The issue, of course, is that in being 'culturally' sensitive, what are the issues being acknowledged, and is there recognition of the full range of socio-economic, political, and biographical arenas that people actually operate in on an everyday basis?

It is not possible to discuss ethnicity and culture, and their interaction with health and illness without considering the embedded-ness of people in historical power relations. As post-war mass migration from Commonwealth countries gained momentum in the 1950s and 1960s, the demographic makeup of Britain assumed major changes. Labour shortages in many industries vital to economic and social growth meant that labourers were initially both welcomed by the government, but shunned by many indigenous White populations due to fear of economic effects. Fear was also of a more emotive and visceral, racialised hue. As Caribbean, Indian, Pakistani, East African, and Chinese people (Ahmad and Bradby 2008; Brah 2006; Craig et al. 2012) arrived in Britain to settle, so the development of changing attitudes became melded into both local and national politics and concerns. As groups settled into both work and life patterns, in addition to experiencing huge amounts of adversity via racism—overt and more implicit—the power of collective organisation and representation took hold, leading to various forms of anti-racism organisation. Sivanandan (1981) writes of the state shifting its emphasis in discourse from structure, power, and racism to ideas of culture, ethnicity, and difference. The 1950s and 1960s heralded a unity among UK 'Black' populations (a political label given to many different groups in Britain at the time struggling to gain acknowledgement of the racism and prejudice experienced), but this unity was seen as a threat. Writers observe that the state disunited this unity, and minority groups were split and disaggregated (Sivanandan 2008). Groups and people became 'ethnically distinct' whereas earlier, they had been 'politically common'. Communities developed 'day centres' and 'special projects', all organised around the notion of distinctive and culturally cohesive communities. Of course, this political 'unity' amongst people from a huge and varied range of backgrounds could not live up to the idealisation it connoted—as Ahmad (1993, 1996) criticises—it was a fiction, since people were already split and divided according to differences other than 'race'.

This wider political point has a relevance for this book since it explores people's experiences of not only the individual and personal illness, but also the wider landscape in terms of connections to community centres, temples, foci of religious and cultural events, and dialogue. While critics of this 'multicultural orthodoxy' point to what Sivanandan calls the commoditisation of cultures (1991), it is these very same units of identity, and locations of religious, cultural, and social interaction which perform highly important functions for mediating peoples' needs. Some critics of this 'identity' politics overlook the efficacy of those provisions at the smaller, localised, and individual level (a point shared by Kelleher 1996). They are partly a result of local projects, and large groups of disadvantaged people rely on them for power, voice, and help. Placing the health and illness states of individuals within the context of a political backdrop provides a wider debate for this study of diabetes experiences. For theorists such as Ahmad (1996), it is impossible to predict the behaviour of an ethnic group on the basis of cultural knowledge, country of origin, or language since there are too many complexities involved. This 'crude multiculturalism' splits groups of people into identifiable chunks for ease of access, and theorists such as Ahmad (1996) debate the value of simplistic and crude versions of multiculturalism when placed against the political power of anti-racism.

Anti-racism, with its roots in the political unity of groups, was able to mobilise and protest against racism—overt and covert—and formed the opposition in terms of major debates of difference. As Brah (1992) summarises, when she writes about the process of 'Ethnicism'—defining experiences in 'culturalist' terms results in ethnic difference becoming the main entity around which social life is experienced. 'Cultural needs' are then defined independently of racism, gender, and sexuality. Wider systems of oppression are effectively masked. However, 'crude antiracism' (Ahmad 1996) is equally ineffective in its ability to generate insights, since it may look at socio-political contexts at the expense of the 'micro' interactions people are involved in. BME people run the risk of becoming solely the effect of racism, and the product of racism, rather than the producers and generators of social action, which involves old and new forms of identity—an idea shared by many other writers (Gunaratnam 2003; Gilroy 2004). Culture is flexible, contested, and shaped by social and structural contexts, generating cultural norms which are flexible guidelines within which behaviour is negotiated.

Conclusion

In this chapter, I have introduced the core substantive themes that will be addressed in this book. The need for conceptualising the often problematic and troubled relationship between health and illness states, and socio-political contexts is paralleled and indeed interlinked with conceptual and theoretical developments in the social sciences. It is not possible to extricate the analysis and critical appreciation of health and illness without a historical and political gaze. Since all acts are political, and all human social practices are characterised by the push and pull of structures and agentive processes, where these power-related tensions materialise in the lives of people who have experienced and in many ways continue to experience the intersectional subjugations of race, class, and gender, a fuller contextualised situated-ness is wholly required.

In the following chapter, I attempt to situate diabetes sociologically in order to contextualise the types of understanding the field has established in explaining the social and culturally mediated health state.

References

Ahmad, W. I. U. (1993). *'Race' and health in contemporary Britain*. Buckingham: Open University Press.

Ahmad, W. I. U. (1996). The trouble with culture. In D. Kelleher & S. Hillier (Eds.), *Researching cultural differences in health* (pp. 190–219). London: Routledge.

Ahmad, W. I. U., & Bradby, H. (2007). Locating ethnicity and health: Exploring concepts and contexts. *Sociology of Health & Illness, 29*(6), 795–810. Available at: http://www.ncbi.nlm.nih.gov/pubmed/17986016. Accessed 13 Nov 2014.

Ahmad, W., & Bradby, H. (2008). Ethnicity and health: Key themes in a developing field. *Current Sociology, 56*(1), 47–56. Available at: http://csi.sagepub.com/cgi/doi/10.1177/0011392107084378. Accessed 13 Nov 2014.

Ahmad, W. I. U., Atkin, K., & Chamba, R. (2000). 'Causing havoc to their children': Parental and professional perspectives on consanguinity and childhood disability. In W. I. U. Ahmad (Ed.), *Ethnicity, disability and chronic illness* (pp. 28–44). Buckingham: Open University Press.

Alexander, C. (2004). Writing race: Ethnography and the imagination of the Asian Gang. In M. Bulmer & J. Solomos (Eds.), *Researching race and racism.* London: Routledge.

Ali, K., Kalra, V. S., & Sayyid, B. (2006). *A postcolonial people – South Asians in Britain.* London: Hurst and Co.

Anionwu, E., & Atkin, K. (2001). *The politics of sickle cell and thalassaemia.* Buckingham: Open University Press.

Barker, M. (1981). *The new racism.* London: Junction Books.

Bauman, Z. (1989). *Modernity and the holocaust.* Cambridge: Polity Press.

Becker, H. S. (1986). *Writing for social scientists.* Chicago: University of Chicago Press.

Bhopal, R. (1997). Is research into ethnicity and health racist, sound, or important science? *British Medical Journal, 314,* 1751.

Bhopal, R. (2006). Race and ethnicity: Responsible use from epidemiological and public health perspectives. *The Journal of Law, Medicine & Ethics, 34 (3),* 500–507, Fall 2006.

Bhopal, R. S. (2007). *Ethnicity, race and health in multicultural societies.* Oxford: Oxford University Press.

Bhopal, R. (2013). A four-stage model explaining the higher risk of type 2 diabetes mellitus in South Asians compared with European populations. *Diabetic Medicine, 30*(1), 35–42. doi:10.1111/dme.12016.

Bloch, A., Neal, S., & Solomos, J. (2013). *Race, multiculture and social policy.* Basingstoke: Palgrave Macmillan.

Bradby, H. (2003). Describing ethnicity in health research. *Ethnicity and Health, 8*(1), 5–13.

Bradby, H. (2012). Review: Race, ethnicity and health: The costs and benefits of conceptualising racism and ethnicity. *Social Science and Medicine, 75,* 955–958.

Brah, A. (1992). Difference, diversity and differentiation. In J. Donald & A. Rattansi (Eds.), *Race, culture and difference*. London: Sage.

Brah, A. (1996). Cartographies of Diaspora: Contesting Identities. Oxon: Routledge.

Brah, A. (2006). The Asian in Britain. In N. Ali, V. S. Kalra, & S. Sayyid (Eds.), *A postcolonial people – South Asians in Britain* (pp. 35–61). London: Hurst and Company.

Chattoo, S., & Atkin, K. (2012). 'Race', ethnicity and social policy: Theoretical concepts and the limitations of current approaches to welfare. In *Understanding 'race' and ethnicity: Theory, history, policy, practice*. Bristol: Policy Press.

Clarke, S. (2006). *Social theory, psychoanalysis and racism*. Basingstoke: Palgrave Macmillan.

Craig, G., Atkin, K., Chatoo, S., & Flynn, R. (Eds.). (2012). *Understanding 'race' and ethnicity: Theory, history, policy, practice*. Bristol: Policy Press.

Dominelli, L. (1988). *Anti-racist social work*. London: Macmillan.

Donovan, J. (1984). Ethnicity and disease: A research overview. *Social Science and Medicine, 19*(7), 663–670.

Fassin, D. (2011). Racialisation: How to do races with bodies. In F. E. Mascia-Lees (Ed.), *Companion to the anthropology of the body and embodiment* (1st ed.). London: Blackwell.

Gilroy, P. (2004). *After empire: Melancholia or convivial culture?* London: Routledge.

Gunaratnam, Y. (2003). *Researching 'race' and ethnicity: Methods, knowledge and power*. London: Sage.

Hall, S. (1992). New ethnicities. In J. Donald & A. Rattanasi (Eds.), *Race, culture and difference*. London: Sage.

Hall, S. (1996). Race: The floating signifier. Lecture at Goldsmiths College, University of London. Transcript available at: https://www.mediaed.org/assets/products/407/transcript_407.pdf. Accessed 20 Oct 2015.

Hilton, B. A., Bottorff, J. L., Johnson, J. L., Venables, L. J., Bilkhu, S., Grewal, S., Popatia, N., Clarke, H., & Sumel, P. (2001). The desi ways: Traditional health practices of South Asian women in Canada. *Health Care for Women International, 22*(6), 553–567.

Jones, J. (1992). *Bad blood: The Tuskagee syphilis experiment* (2nd ed.). New York: The Free Press.

Kelleher, D. (1996). A defence of the use of terms 'ethnicity' and 'culture'. In D. Kelleher & S. Hillier (Eds.), *Researching cultural differences in health* (pp. 69–90). London: Routledge.

Keval, H. (2015). Risky cultures to risky genes: The racialised discursive construction of South Asian genetic diabetes risk. *New Genetics and Society*. doi:10.1080/14636778.2015.1036155.

Krieger, N. (1994). Epidemiology and the web of causation: Has anyone seen the spider? *Social Science and Medicine, 39*, 887–903.

Krieger, N., Smith, K., Naishadham, D., Harman, C., & Barbeau, E. M. (2005). Experiences of discrimination: Validity and reliability of a self-report measure for population health research on racism and health. *Social Science & Medicine, 61*(7), 1576e1596.

Lambert, H., & Sevak, M. (1996). Is cultural difference a useful concept? Perceptions of health and sources of ill health among Londoners of South Asian origin. In D. Kelleher & S. Hillier (Eds.), *Researching cultural differences in health*. London: Routledge.

Lawton, J., Peel, E., Parry, O., Araoza, G., & Douglas, M. (2005). Lay perceptions of type 2 diabetes in Scotland: Bringing health services back in. *Social Science & Medicine, 60*, 1423–1435.

Lentin, A. (2014). Postracial silences the othering of race in Europe. In W. D. Hund & A. Lentin (Eds.), *Racism and sociology* (pp. 1–35). Berlin: Lit.

Littlewood, R., & Lipsedge, M. (1989). *Aliens and alienists. Ethnic minorities and psychiatry*. London: Unwin Hyman.

Malik, K. (1996). *The meaning of race: Race history and culture in Western society*. London: Macmillan Press/New York University Press.

Malik, K. (2009). The new language of diversity. Race: Science's Last Taboo, pp. 1–5. 2009 Channel Four Television Corporation. Available at: http://www.channel4.com/explore/raceandscience/

Montoya, M. J. (2011). *Making the Mexican diabetic: Race, science, and the genetics of inequality*. London: University of California Press.

Nagel, J. (1994). Constructing ethnicity: Creating and recreating ethnic identity and culture. *Social Problems, 41*(1), 152–176.

Nazroo, J. (1997). *The health of Britain's ethnic minorities: Findings from a national survey*. London: Policy Studies Institute.

Nazroo, J. Y. (2003). The structuring of ethnic inequalities in health: Economic position, racial discrimination, and racism. *American Journal of Public Health, 93*(2), 277–284. Available at: http://ajph.aphapublications.org/doi/abs/10.2105/AJPH.93.2.277.

Nazroo, J., & Karlsen, S. (2002). Agency and structure: The impact of ethnic identity and racism on the health of ethnic minority people. *Sociology of Health & Illness, 24*(1), 1–20.

Rocheron, Y. (1988). The Asian mother and baby campaign: The construction of ethnic minorities health needs. *Critical Social Policy, 22*, 4–23.

Said, E. (1977). *Orientalism*. London: Penguin.

Sheldon, T., & Parker, H. (1992). Race and ethnicity in health research. *Journal of Public Health Medicine, 14*(2), 104–110.

Sivanandan, A. (1981). From resistance to rebellion: Asian and Afro-Caribbean struggles in Britain. *Race & Class, 23*(2–3), 111–152. Available at: http://rac.sagepub.com/cgi/doi/10.1177/030639688102300202. Accessed 13 Nov 2014.

Sivanandan, A. (1991). *'Black struggles against racism' in centre for education and training in social work anti-racist social work education: Setting the context for change*. London: CCETSW.

Sivanandan, A. (2008). *Catching history on the wing – Race culture and globalisation*. London: Pluto Press.

Smaje, C. (1995). *Health, 'race' and ethnicity: Making sense of the evidence*. London: The King's Fund.

Smaje, C. (1996). The ethnic patterning of health: New directions for theory and research. *Sociology of Health and Illness, 18*(2), 139–171.

Smaje, C. (2000). Race, ethnicity, and health. In C. E. Bird, P. Conrad, & A. M. Fremont (Eds.), *Handbook of medical sociology*. Englewood Cliffs: Prentice Hall.

Stubbs, P. (1993). Ethnically sensitive' or 'anti-racist'? Models for research and service delivery. In W. I. U. Ahmad (Ed.), *'Race' and health in contemporary Britain*. Buckingham: Open University Press.

Taylor, P. (2013). *Race*. Cambridge: Polity Press.

Wohland, P., Rees, P., Nazroo, J., & Jagger, C. (2014). Inequalities in healthy life expectancy between ethnic groups in England and Wales in 2001. *Ethnicity & Health*. doi:10.1080/13557858.2014.921892.

3

Situating the South Asian Diabetic Risk

In the last chapter, I focused on developing an understanding of how ethnicity, culture, and race are conceptualised in both research and practice, within academic and interventionist circles. The way in which patterns and discussions of risk generate specific, contemporary meanings of race/ethnicity and risk is an important, discursive, and symbolic marker. It points to both the specifics of epistemological underpinnings and the long, related history of biological race-thinking, but also takes us into wider, socio-cultural identifications of how race and ethnicity, minority populations, and health have become mutually intertwined.

In this chapter, I first define and discuss the nature of diabetes, then explore some experiential medical sociological and anthropological literature in order to then situate the experience of diabetes in a more nuanced fashion. Previous chapters have contextualised BME experiences of health and illness within the wider socio-structural context of racialised health inequalities. These studies and writings, amongst others, have firmly established these racialised patterns. Given that the multiple strands of this book converge on the experience of people with diabetes, it is apposite to begin with the everyday knowledge and ideas of people, which inform their practices, and

© The Editor(s) (if applicable) and The Author(s) 2016
H. Keval, *Health, Ethnicity and Diabetes*,
DOI 10.1057/978-1-137-45703-5_3

importantly, have become the focus of many health service provider–user interrelations. Staying within the foci of experience, this chapter moves onto the role of biography, and its importance in exploring diabetes, to show that the constructions of South Asian diabetes discourse, as they orbit around notions of passivity and 'non-compliance', are countered by *how people use their biographical expertise*. The role of biography, therefore, becomes integral to understanding lay knowledge claims and constructions. The chapter then explores the epidemiological status of diabetes worldwide and nationally so that a more detailed picture is rendered. The aim, however, is not just to describe and report these figures but also to situate them within a wider discursive framework. I start with some definitional discussions regarding diabetes.

Defining Diabetes

Diabetes mellitus is a disease which affects the proper functioning of the body's glucose levels. Insulin, a hormone normally naturally created by the pancreas, is released into the bloodstream and regulates the levels of glucose in the blood. Glucose, a type of blood sugar which is vital for the body to transform into energy and various other uses, is usually maintained by the insulin at a level which is optimal for the body's functioning. When food is eaten, the body changes most of the food intake into glucose. The blood then carries the glucose to various cells in the body, to perform the pre-programmed instructions held in the genetic code. The glucose needs insulin to get into the body cells. In a diabetic patient, either the pancreas does not create enough insulin (or fails completely) or there is enough resistance to the insulin (in the form of receptor cells in body tissues failing to utilise the insulin that is produced) to cause a malfunction, and this can lead to many complications, including kidney failure, neuropathology, and retinopathy, and to death (Rubin 2001).

Types of Diabetes

There are various types of diabetes, but the two types which are the focus of much research are type 1 and type 2. There are other types of diabetes, which are features of particular global and socio-political-economic conditions (famine-related) or particular biomedical conditions (such as gestational diabetes, common during pregnancy)—these are not the focus of this study. Type 1 diabetes is an insulin-dependent condition (IDDM—Insulin-Dependent Diabetes Mellitus), which means that the individual's body depends on an external source of insulin to regulate glucose levels. This condition is perceived to be serious in terms of prognosis, treatment, effects on the body's functions, and related life expectancy. Type 1 diabetes appears when the pancreas produces little or no insulin, causing the glucose levels in the blood to be without control. A dysfunction in insulin production can cause a variety of problems, including fat and muscle formation enhanced by insulin, storage of glucose, and protein breakdown prevention. Type 1 is an auto-immune disease, whereby the insulin-producing cells (beta cells) are destroyed by the body itself. Typical treatment is through a combination of medication, insulin (made from various sources, usually animal [pig] based), diet, and exercise regimes. Type 2 diabetes, also known as non-insulin-dependent diabetes mellitus (NIDDM), is the more common variety of diabetes. This condition is characterised by an insulin resistance syndrome which makes the processing of insulin and maintenance of glucose difficult. This condition is also known as Mature Onset Diabetes, as it usually appears or is diagnosed in later life, at around the age of 40. The typical treatment for the condition is a regime of medication (usually tablets), nutritional and diet modification, exercise, and the maintenance of lowered fat levels in the body (since increased body fat and obesity are said to cause deterioration of the condition). Although there is insulin being produced, the body resists the normal functioning of insulin—the insulin resistance syndrome—which can then lead to type 2 diabetes. In terms of signs and symptoms, there are a number of commonalities between the two types, which become a crucial part of the patient's experiential knowledge base. Fatigue, frequent urination, and thirst are common to both, but the differences are important. Type 2 symptoms also include blurred vision, slow healing of infections, numbness in extreme limbs, heart disease, and obesity.

A 'New' Condition?

Whilst the contemporary research, policy, and public awareness of the 'diabetes time bomb' (a quick internet search of this phrase yields plentiful media reporting, as does adding the term 'South Asian') appears to be a recent emergence, in tandem with changes in post-industrial and globalised sedentary life, diabetes itself has a longer history. The term 'diabetes mellitus' is a Greco-Latin term sourced in their respective histories. The Romans found that sometimes urine would be sweet tasting—it tasted *mellitus* (Latin for 'sweet'). Before this, records from Greek history noted that sometimes, people with this sweet urine produced fluids almost immediately, like a siphon, and hence, called this condition *diabetes* (Latin for 'siphon', Rubin 2001). This early definition of the physical ailment was not limited to early Greek civilisation, as Ancient Hindu texts as early as 1000 BC, in recorded observations similar to that of the Romans much later, recall ants swarming near a spot of urine, indicating *Madhumeha* ('honey urine'), which, if neglected, could finally lead to *Prameha* (Diabetes). Official Indian medical treatises formed in 600 AD define clearly the condition of diabetes mellitus or Prameha (Subbulakshmi and Naik 2001), suggesting that while diabetes has moved to a worldwide health agenda in modern times, it also has a long cultural history.

Complications

One of the many primary concerns for diabetes sufferers (types 1 and 2) is the range of complications and effects of the condition on the human body. Life expectancies for people suffering from diabetes are also reduced. For type 1 sufferers, 20 years are taken off the average life span, while for type 2, the life duration is reduced by 10 years, not including those serious, and sometimes fatal, complications of eye disease, renal failure, and limb extremity neuropathology (Diabetes UK 2013). Although I will avoid making substantial comments on the physiological nature of the complication, it is prudent to touch upon no less because of the differential rates at which people present with complications, but also since treatment and complications of diabetes costs £8.8 billion a year (Hex et al. 2012). Current data indicates a stark echo of historical data trends—that BME communities and South Asians, in particular, suffer higher rates of complications (Gholap et al. 2011; Chowdhury and Lasker 2002). Both type 1 and 2 diabetics run a risk of developing a certain number of established complications. Kidney problems, eyesight impairment, peripheral nerve damage of the extremities, and autonomous nerve system problems are all commonly reported problems. Whilst biomedical and genetic science has progressed considerably from the early days of diabetes, there is still no way of definitely avoiding these complications. The universal point which emanates from nearly all information and guidance sources (including the National Institute for Health Care and Excellence (NICE), Department of Health, Diabetes UK, International Diabetes Federation, World Health Organisation, and South Asian Health Foundation) is to monitor blood glucose levels, maintain normalcy according to a predefined level, and implement strategies of insulin level change. Diet, exercise, education, and professional health advice are still regarded as the only methods of keeping the illness under some control.

Lay Health Experiences

The wide-ranging research into what has come to be known as 'lay' experiences (Calnan 1987; Prior 2003; Lawton 2003) of health and illness is extensive and diverse, dealing with class and socio-economic contexts (d'Houtard and Field 1984; Popay et al. 1998), a variety of chronic illnesses (Bury 1982; Williams 1984; Anderson and Bury 1988), and gender (Blaxter 1983), to name a small number. Lay ideas have been deemed central to our understanding of the social positioning and embeddedness of health and illness states, and point us in the direction of contextual recognition of explanations for social phenomena. Where once non-medical citizens were simply 'wrong' if their ideas were different from the professional arena's ideas, lay health ideas are now given legitimacy. Prior (2003) discusses the legitimation crises in the professions as resulting in more partnership with citizens regarding medical healthcare, while Turner (2001) points to changes in knowledge status and ownership. As established convention in this field indicates, lay ideas are not simply watered-down versions of medical knowledge, but rather shaped, structured, and influenced by biographies and histories. If lay ideas are as Lambert and Sevak (1996) suggest, embedded within cultural constructs and individual histories, then there is a conceptual and empirical need for a more nuanced recognition of what these cultural and social contexts are, when played out alongside biographical experiences. A straightforward rendering of an account as a lay account is, therefore, not sufficient for the purposes of this research.

As Prior (2003) argues, there is a wealth of information lay people have about their bodies. These knowledge frameworks are about their experiences of the condition and the impact of pain and disruption on their lives. But they are rarely professionals with a competency in technical medical arenas, and for this reason, Prior (2003) warns against the use of the term 'lay expert'. Though this sounds like a blow to the lay health frameworks important in the sociology of health and illness, I support this vigilance—for two reasons. First, there are semantic, conceptual, and practical implications of being an 'expert' and these are the markers that differentiate one from having a lay role. Second, to use the term 'lay expert' is to invite the objective/subjective dichotomy, and this is too easily transposed to the 'correct/incorrect' equation. Shaw and Gould (2001) call to move away from the focus on lay health 'beliefs' and to concentrate more on the accounts people produce—a point echoing earlier suggestions by Radley and Billig (1996)—is perhaps more useful than focusing on semantics. As Prior states, people are 'expertly experiential' (2003: 54), but we should not confuse the two separate areas of technical medical expertise and lay participation and consultation in medical matters.

The Role of Biography

In the last few decades there have been a number of studies which have changed the way illness has been regarded by social scientists (see Lawton 2003). There are a number of prominent biographical-themed sociologies, which help us to understand the relevance of biography in health and illness. Bury's 'biographical disruption' (1983), which focuses on the way that an illness can be a major disruption in life—drawing on Giddens' (1991) work to articulate the critical nature of the disruption—is useful here. The ontological 'tear' which occurs during a chronic illness causes a crucial shift in a person's biography and self-concept. The multilayered nature of this shift leads to a reappraisal of ones' life trajectory in psychological, emotional, and physical/material realms. The relevance of this 'disruption'-focused schema to this study is obvious—the onset of later diagnosed diabetes (type 2) can have a major effect on the individual with the illness, and affect many aspects of their daily operation. Type 2 diabetes is a disease which, although carrying many serious psycho-social impacts, is also a condition which can be managed with great success (as is the case with insulin-dependent diabetes or type 1). We can, however, raise some useful questions: how do these normatively prescribed sociological identifications of 'experience' figure in those health and illness situations which are doubly impacted by illness and racialised experiences? How does a biography that may be disrupted, or indeed, that requires *continuity work:* (a) deal with these demands in the face of multiple life events, and (b) actively use cultural and ethnic identity to negotiate this landscape? What I am exploring in this book is the disruption, and perhaps, those ongoing experiences of loss of self (Charmaz 1983), but more importantly, the way in which cultural, biographical, social resources are constantly utilised to negotiate difficulties. People may mobilise resources, maintain relationships and activities, and as Rajaram asserts, emphasise the role of stigma, through the process of 'biographical reconstruction… strive(s) to maintain a positive sense of self…' (1997: 283). The resultant change in 'self' is explored by Charmaz (1983), who focuses on how chronically ill people may lose a sense of 'self'. Self-images are seen to be gradually destroyed, without any new, positive, and valued ones taking their place. As Lawton (2003) summarises, Charmaz advances our understanding in two main ways. First, we are given a perspective of illness in an everyday context, rather than a narrow medical view, and second, the multifaceted nature of the illness is discussed—problems with self-identity in one area lead to problems in other areas. The value of this 'loss of self' approach is substantial for approaching the way diabetic patients might view themselves, their illness, and their life, within the context of their condition. As other aspects of their lives are also affected by the nutrition, medication, physical, symptomatic, and social changes they experience, so would we also expect a change in identity. What is less researched and explored in contemporary research is how these interacting, over-laid, and shifting senses of identity, as reflected in ethno-cultural and ethno-religious contexts, are related to the understanding of diabetes.

In order to pursue some notion of what I have called the 'discursive construction of South Asian diabetes risk', we need to have a sense of what official agencies are reporting in diabetes trends. The 'risk package' is a collection of concepts, methodologies, theories, and interventions, generated, driven, and maintained by government (e.g. Department for Health, NICE) and non-government (Diabetes UK, International Diabetes Federation) agencies. The 'package' (part of what Montoya (2011) calls the 'diabetes enterprise') is also connected to, maintained, and developed with academic agencies carrying out research cutting across the traditional academia–practice divide. This section, therefore, in one sense 'performs' the epidemiological representations of diabetes prevalence and incidence, but utilises a critical gaze by situating this data firmly within the nexus of discursive constructions. Montoya (2011) suggests it is not that there *isn't* a relationship between patterns of disease and groups; there clearly is. The problem lies with how this relationship is manifested in the South Asian diabetes 'package', mobilising stereotypes, tropes, and misconceptualisations of culture and difference.

What's in a Name?

There is a need to view diabetes health science discourse from this critical perspective, and Hedgecoe's sociology of scientific knowledge applied to the area of genetics and society (Hedgecoe 2001, 2002) is most useful. In his diabetes-specific work, his approach reveals the contingent nature of the scientific process, especially the dynamics of labelling conditions. Whilst I do not intend to labour on this point nor explore this in depth, it serves to spell out the ways in which meaning-making in scientific and biomedical research enterprises involves a variety of negotiated decisions, themselves deeply enmeshed in complex networks of compromise-requiring actions. The naming process of diabetes as 'type 1' and 'type 2' (Hedgecoe 2002) was far from being a straightforward result of neutral and objective descriptive decisions. Rather, it emerges as the meeting point of both scientific subject-related conceptualisations, and importantly, the subtle and politically charged process of power relations. This then shows us that a condition we *know* to be accepted as a specific disease entity, represented in epidemiological data, research enterprises, government reports, guidance, and policy, is also one which is 'performed' to be, in many ways, the epitome of a fixed, unchanging, disease entity. The stability of the entity is what generates confidence in producers and consumers of this package of ideas, and thus, diabetes—type 1 or type 2—when used in conjunction with the mobilisation of other 'fixed' representations of difference. These 'imaginings' of how identities of difference can *determine* health are situated in the long and myopic history of how 'minorities' are processed generally (Atkin 2006).

Given the established positivist empirical model of observing, counting, and reporting has now been established as also being a constructed process (Bhopal 2007), it is of no surprise that how specific groups of people in society become categorised, diagnosed, counted, and treated can be seen as a contingent, dynamic, and discursively constructed series of events. In Foucauldian terms, the creation, maintenance, and application of diagnostic categories holds a wealth of power relations. The way in which diabetes has been investigated is, as Hedgecoe (2002) has pointed out, subject to discursive bending and shaping. Hedgecoe's work shows how science and knowledge mobilise various power relations so that particular forms of representation take precedence over others. Diabetes is one of many conditions which are categorically, scientifically, and empirically contingent on the way science-knowledge-making agents can mediate particular versions of knowledge. Bioscience, however, is not alone in this trend, since the South Asian diabetes 'risk package' has been discursively situated within sociological debates. Some of this work rests upon health service access and take-up evaluations, the experiential universe of the condition, and its impacts on one's personal, cultural, and ethnic identity. Other health and social science-flavoured work has emphasised the very same cultural or group deviance which I discussed in the last chapter. North American anthropological accounts have, by far, been the most nuanced, rich, and critically insightful analyses of the overall complexity of racial health discourses (e.g. Ferreira and Lang 2006; Scheper-Hughes 2006; Farmer 2004). The UK medical sociology arena, it appears, has some catching up to do. The point I am making is that all intellectual, knowledge-building exercises are rooted in specific and particular ground, and this ground often is saturated with already extant visible and invisible racial meanings. British medical sociology has been accused of ignoring these crucial debates, with some key authors and researchers in this area, such as Ahmad (1992), arguing that sociology had completely ignored its responsibility to reflect the ethnic and religious diversity that was a clear backdrop to medical sociological work.

Although there has been substantial progress in the quantity and variation of research involving ethnicity in health, diabetes has proved to be a case where both the academy and policy agencies appear to have consensus on what direction they need to move forward in. The direction is, on the one hand, laudable, since it speaks to the intuitive sense of ethical responsibility that emerges from community-based intervention programmes, audits of service access, and constant research reporting of various diabetes management-based programmes. These are located both nationally in terms of official government policy, and situated within more localised initiatives. There is another side to this, however, and it is this alternative, but parallel, version of diabetes risk which concerns this book. The emerging picture rendered by decades of epidemiological surveys, biomedical research, health service evaluations and audits, and 'diversity' health research, its usefulness notwithstanding, is one imbued, and inundated, with racial meanings. The very way in which race, ethnicity, and culture—indeed, *difference itself*—is conceptualised is *necessarily* mediated, buffered, and shaped by historical legacies of migration, colonial connections, and immigration. I argue that whilst there are researchers, authors, and work in existence which indeed make this discourse central for moving forward in contemporary multicultural and diverse health arenas, both the social science and policy work has left the discursive, 'raciological' (Gilroy 2012) landscape relatively untouched. My aim, in this section, is therefore to situate the epidemiological, lifestyle and cultural discursive meaning-making against a critical gaze.

Misattributions of Causality

I do not refer to the oft-cited South Asian diabetes picture as the 'Asian diabetes time bomb' to trivialise the very serious nature of the condition, or undermine the valiant and consistent efforts of the many agencies involved in collecting the data. Rather, the aim is to generate some understanding of differential rates, experiences, access to services and treatment/recovery rates. I refer to it as the 'time bomb' because the media focus has consistently been on the differential rates of diabetes, and subsequently, moved within their accounts to explanations centring on culture, lifestyle, and diet. The explicit absence of race-based discourse and persistent inclusion of ethnic and cultural notions within media treatment are only reinforced by the underlying assumption that *the presence of the differential numbers must mean the difference is racial.* As I point out in the previous chapter, one does not necessarily imply the other; this becomes an example of misconceptualisation of health, ethnicity, and group membership, and misattribution of causality. 'Race' or 'ethnicity' by itself does not cause diabetes. As Happe (2013), utilising Lewontin's (1991) work, reminds us that in the case of cancer,

> [a]sbestos and cotton lint fibres are not causes of cancer. They are the agents of social causes, of social formations that determine the nature of our productive and consumptive lives…it is only through the changes to those social forces that we can get to the root of problems in health. (Lewontin 1991, cited in Happe)

South Asian diabetes is not the result of racial, ethnic, or cultural difference. By and large, the way in which the South Asian diabetes 'high risk package' is represented in policy, practice, and debate (excluding critical sociology and anthropology) is overwhelmingly focused on biological, cultural, and now, genetically inflected explanations.

I have already alluded to the comparative nature of epidemiologically-based concerns in the health of minority populations, invoking long-established critical authors such as Ahmad (1993). The way in which health concerns often become the subject of raised anxiety, and then, official focus is through comparisons to data on 'White' counterparts. This, as I have explained, has difficulties attached to it—namely, the conceptualisation of group membership based entirely on constructed, historical catego-ries of difference, and the fact that comparing 'BME' groups to 'White' groups—the latter being the population standard against which the 'oth-ers' are measured—is highly problematic in its assumption of normative ideals. What characteristic could it be that could constitute the grouping 'South Asian' (or 'White', for that matter) to a sufficient extent to ignore the vast range of differences within the group, in relation to country of ori-gin, language, religion/faith, socio-economic status, generational position, geographical location, number of years/generations in the UK, material position pre-migration to the UK, and experiences of trauma and stress? (Nazroo 2003) The point is that group identities—ethno-religious, cul-tural, or otherwise—cannot *cause* illness. The multiple shifting meanings attached to difference, and how these are treated in concentric circles of economic influence within a polity, become central to this discussion. This does not devalue health interventions where they are most needed, but rather, encourages cognisance of the complexities in this arena. Developing 'strategies' to tackle the extant and historical 'minority health issues' does not necessarily constitute *counter-'race-thinking'*. It can be a mutually exclu-sive damaging and derogative relationship that emerges in health interven-tions if conceptualisations of difference have not been thought through critically. Having made these points, I now turn to what the epidemiology indicators can tell us about the global picture of diabetes.

Trends, Patterns, and the Politics of Counting: The Worldwide and UK Picture

There are an estimated 382 million people worldwide with the disease (IDF 2013). Nearly 5 million deaths in 2012 alone were accountable to diabetes, and the majority of these were in low-income countries (WHO

2013). The World Health Organisation predicts that, by 2030, diabetes will be the seventh leading cause of global fatalities (WHO 2013). While people in what we might define as 'industrialised' and 'developed' countries carry a massive burden of the illness, with 3.2 million currently in the UK, with a projected rise to 5 million by 2025, and America hosting over 25 million (IDF 2013), other countries carry an even larger burden (IDF 2013). India, China, and the Western Pacific states have massively accelerating rates of diabetes and much of the increase has been explained by the condition's nominal status as a 'lifestyle affliction'. The IDF emphasises that there is a widely held misconception that diabetes is a 'disease of the wealthy' (2013: 7) and point out that 80 % of diabetics live in countries with low-to-middle income. There is a research consensus that as societies make the transition from a traditional to a more 'complex', industrialised, modern, and leisure-driven one, the attending impacts on people's physiology take their toll. In short, modern sedentary and calorie-rich lifestyles, especially for those groups who have only recently 'modernised', have the greatest impact on health.

The South Asian Picture

From the outer concentric circles of worldwide figures and a generalised national picture of prevalence, we can move to some specific rates of diabetes. It should be noted that here, these figures are not contested for their accuracy. Rather, they become a topic of interest because of their scientific 'immutability'. Epidemiological, quantitative evidence forms part of a larger representational system of numbers, categories, ideas, and has an impact on both policy and people. This is fairly self-evident, as changes in the rates would correspond to changes in the various related components of health provision. However, at the heart of this 'immutability' is also a conceptual framework, which characterises difference in specific, countable ways. It seems fairly logical to argue that if we can't count how many people are ill, then we can't help improve their health or the vital services that can be put in place for them. However, the machinery of epidemiology is not driven by value-free and neutral scientific calculation, but is also a social, political, and culturally located constellation of decisions. How epidemics come to discursively have symbolic power is worth exploring (Rock 2003). While my aim in this book is not particularly to focus on the social construction of epidemiological science, given the early warnings framed by critical authors in this area, it appears prudent to maintain critical vigilance.

There is a wide variety of information sources on the 'South Asian diabetes risk'—from research articles in peer-reviewed publications, non-governmental organisations, official government agencies, through to media outlets which periodically warn of diabetes epidemics and 'time bombs'. Here, I utilise a number of sources so that we can at least start to explore the extent of the diagnosed condition of diabetes within a given population, maintaining vigilance against many of the simplistic conceptualisations that are generated, mobilised, and then used in health service delivery.

The patterns that we find now in the epidemiology of South Asian diabetes were emergent in the 1980s in an area of London—Southall (Bhopal 2013; Nagi 2004). These patterns showed large differences between White Europeans and South Asian groups. The general trend since then has been to confirm this finding, with rates quoted generally as between five and eight times higher in South Asian groups than in White populations (see Gholap 2011; Simmons et al. 1992; Wild and Chaturvedi 2009; D'Costa et al. 2000). People of South Asian origin are exposed to an increased risk of diabetes (Davies 1999) and present with diabetes at a younger age than Caucasians (McKeigue and Marmot 1988). This finding is supported by other studies, which indicate a three–five times higher risk amongst African-Caribbean and South Asian populations (Davey Smith et al. 2002). Similarly, earlier studies, such as the Health Survey for England (1999), showed the highest diabetes prevalence rates among Bangladeshis (10.6 %), although the other South Asian groups also showed high rates (Pakistanis 8.7 %, Indians 7.7 %). The highest age-standardised rates of diabetes were found among South Asian men and women: in particular, Pakistanis and Bangladeshis of both sexes showed rates over five times higher than the general population. Indian men and women were almost three times as likely as the general population to report diabetes. All of these incidence and prevalence rates, are, of course, further complicated by the relationship to cardiovascular diseases (CVD) (which include coronary heart disease and stroke) (Gholap 2011; UKPDS 1998). South Asian people are more at risk of developing these associated diseases, especially since epidemiology indicates that both type 2 diabetes and CVD are more likely to develop earlier in this group than in others (Oldroyd et al. 2005).

Interestingly, while there appears to be a 'wall' of conclusive, extensive evidence to bolster the general scientific finding of South Asian diabetes risk, Wild and Farouhi (2009) critique the parallel lack of population-based evidence. Since epidemiological evidence often does not distinguish between type 1 and type 2, accurate information is difficult to establish, and as the authors above point out, hospital admission and medical records in relation to diabetes and ethnicity are not always accurately represented. Firm foundations of these heightened risks come from bringing together many different studies in a variety of locations throughout the UK (themselves crucial to gaining a better picture of health statuses in minority groups). Data from studies in Coventry, Southall, London, Newcastle, and Manchester have been used to generate population-based estimates of diabetes, which resulted in the generally accepted figure of 'four- to six-fold higher prevalence in South Asian people compared with Europeans' (Wild and Farouhi 2009: 13). This indicates that, as the South Asian Health Foundation (2009) has strongly asserted, more focused and better conceptualised research needs to take place. Importantly, the wall of evidence previously perceived about the South Asian 'time bomb' is itself a conglomeration of findings, scientific interpretations, and effectively, an 'epidemiological bricolage' whose impact is far-ranging in terms of how people are written into the discursive constructions of diabetic risk.

Diabetes is a feature of the South Asian population, both in the UK and in India. North American researchers have carried out in-depth research into the interaction between the environment and ethnic predisposition to type 2 diabetes (Abate and Chandalia 2003). This hugely complex picture involves processes of urbanisation and Westernisation, and their effects on particular ethnic groupings. For example, in rural areas of India, there is a diabetes prevalence of 2 %. In urban areas, this increases to 8 %. In the CURES (Chennai Urban Rural Epidemiology Study 2003) study, 22.3 % of the population was defined as obese (the sample size was 26,000), with obesity increasing with monthly income (Deepa et al. 2003)—a correlation of importance in the context of diabetes perceived globally as a disease of affluence, but also interesting in its contrast to the IDF estimates. Similarly, for those who have migrated to Europe or other 'Westernised' countries, the prevalence again increases to four times higher than those in India (Dowse et al. 1990; McKeigue et al. 1989). This impact of global human movement occurs across many different ethnic groupings, as Abate and Chandalia (2003) show, but there is also another issue; different groups may appear to have different predispositions when faced with similar environments. The public health implications are potentially substantial if certain groups of people are more susceptible than others to diabetes. These predispositions are important because how they are understood and used has an impact on how diabetes becomes embedded in health science discourse.

In response to such questions and issues raised about the epidemiological convenience of these patterns, a range of authors situate diabetes not only within its social and cultural contexts but also firmly within a political economical arena. Mendenhall et al. (2010: 221) see the 'disease of modernisation' as holding important information that can often be missed by simply comparing rates across populations. As Mendenhall argues, citing Mokdad et al. (2001), the prevalence and distribution of diabetes are closely correlated to economic development, and while places such as North America have higher rates of diabetes than, for example, economically depressed regions, such as sub-Saharan Africa, even within wealthy regions, people experiencing poverty are disproportionately affected.

There are other factors, such as stresses of various kinds, that have been known to be associated with prevalence of type 2 diabetes (Mooy et al. 2000). Migration and the related exposure to different cultural, social, political, and linguistic factors may cause inordinate amounts of stress. The South Asian population in the UK has been the subject of many studies, which highlight the cross-cultural problems of living in a host country with problematic climate (Ballard 1994; Visram 2002; Hill 1969; Hiro 1992). Such theories propose either that the migration has such a stressful effect on the migrant that their health is effected or that the natural selection involved in voluntary migration entails a 'healthy migrant' factor. Neither of these is sufficient in explaining the process of health status negotiation, and this is one of the major themes explored in this book.

While we have seen above that prevalence and incidence rates can often be identified as the starting points to thinking about research in the relationship between diabetes and ethnicity, they also need to be identified as a contestable, debateable, constructed set of processes. Epidemiology itself is not simply the counting of existing cases and new cases of disease over time, but in the tradition of the sociology of knowledge, a far more complex, nuanced, and processual nexus of changing, and values-driven dynamics. As Nancy Krieger (2001) identifies, there is an intimate relationship between population patterns of good and bad health, deprivation and privilege, cause and effect, and the perceived actions required to ameliorate poor health. Therefore, the vast amount of social epidemiological information that is now available regarding, for example, South Asian diabetes begins to take on a reified state. This becomes fixed conceptually, but crucially, also dictates terms of action taken to remedy the 'high risk'.

Conclusion

Wherever one looks for information regarding diabetes in the South Asian grouping, one is faced with a representational simulacra, perhaps a form of social epidemiological branding. In this case, the statistical finding of higher rates—in other words, the 'risk package' I alluded to earlier—takes on a metonymic significance. The constituent parts of the metonym then extend to causal factors—lifestyle, diet, culture, and genetics—finally resting on the treatment of not only the condition but also whatever faults or deviances may lie with the groups in question. Difference itself becomes an explanation for the disorder. In the following chapter, I explore these multiple discursive constructions of lifestyle and genetic risk as a way of broadening the view of 'ethnic' diabetes.

References

Abate, N., & Chandalia, M. (2003). The impact of ethnicity on type 2 diabetes. *Journal of Diabetes and Its Complications, 17*, 39–58.

Ahmad, W. I. U. (1992). Is medical sociology an ostrich? Reflections on 'race' and the sociology of health. *Medical Sociology News, 17*(2), 16–21.

Ahmad, W. I. U. (1993). *'Race' and health in contemporary Britain*. Buckingham: Open University Press.

Anderson, R., & Bury, M. (1988). *Living with chronic illness: The experience of patients and their families*. London: Unwin Hyman.

Atkin, K. (2006). Health care and Br Asians: Making sense of policy and practice. In K. Ali, V. S. Kalra, & B. Sayyid (Eds.), *A postcolonial people – South Asians in Britain*. London: Hurst and Co.

Ballard, R. (1994). *Desh Pardesh: The South Asian presence in Britain*. London: Hurst.

Bhopal, R. S. (2007). *Ethnicity, race and health in multicultural societies*. Oxford: Oxford University Press.

Bhopal, R. (2013). A four-stage model explaining the higher risk of type 2 diabetes mellitus in South Asians compared with European populations. *Diabetic Medicine, 30*(1), 35–42. doi:10.1111/dme.12016.

Blaxter, M. (1983). The causes of disease: Women talking. *Social Science and Medicine, 17*, 59–69.

Bury, M. (1982). Chronic illness as biographical disruption. *Sociology of Health and Illness, 4*, 167–182.

Calnan, M. (1987). *Health and illness: The lay perspective*. London: Tavistock.

Charmaz, K. (1983). Loss of self: A fundamental form of suffering in the chronically ill. *Sociology of Health and Illness, 5*, 168–195.

Chowdhury, T. A., & Lasker, S. S. (2002). Complications and cardiovascular risk factors in South Asians and Europeans with early onset type 2 diabetes. *Quarterly Journal of Medicine, 95*, 241–246.

Davey Smith, G., Chaturvedi, N., Harding, S., Nazroo, J., & Williams, R. (2002). Ethnic inequalities in health: A review of UK epidemiological evidence. In S. Sarah Nettleton & U. Gustavson (Eds.), *The sociology of health and illness reader* (pp. 256–257). Cambridge: Polity.

Davies, M. J. (1999). Screening for type 2 diabetes mellitus in the UK Indo-Asian population. *Diabetic Medicine, 16*, 131–137.

Davies, M. J., Yates, T., & Khunti, K. (2009). Prevention of type 2 diabetes. In K. Khunti, S. Kumar, & J. Brodie (Eds.), *Diabetes UK and South Asian Health Foundation recommendations on diabetes research priorities for British South Asians*. London: Diabetes UK.

D'Costa, F. D., Samanta, A., & Burden, A. C. (2000). Epidemiology of diabetes in UK Asians: A review. *Practical Diabetes, 8*, 64–66.

Deepa, M., Pradeepa, R., Rema, M., Mohan, A., Deepa, R., Shanthirani, S., & Mohan, V. (2003). 'The Chennai Urban Rural Epidemiology Study (CURES) – Study design and methodology' (urban component) (CURES – 1). *Journal of Association of Physicians of India, 51*, 862–870.

Department of Health. (1999). *Health survey for England – The health of minority ethnic groups.* London: The Stationery Office.

d'Houtard, A., & Field, M. G. (1984). The image of health: Variations in perception by social class in a French population. *Sociology of Health and Illness, 6,* 30–60.

Dowse, G. K., Gareeboo, H., Zimmett, P. Z., Alberti, K. G., Tuomelehto, J., Fareed, D., Brissonnette, L. G., & Finch, C. F. (1990). High prevalence of NIDDM and impaired glucose tolerance in Indian, Creole, and Chinese Mauritians, Mauritius Non-communicable Disease Study Group. *Diabetes, 39*(3), 390–396.

Diabet Med. 2013 Jul;29(7):855-62. doi: 10.1111/j.1464-5491.2012.03698.x. Estimating the current and future costs of Type 1 and Type 2 diabetes in the UK, including direct health costs and indirect societal and productivity costs.

Farmer, P. (2004). An anthropology of structural violence. *Current Anthropology, 45*(3), 305–317.

Ferreira, M., & Lang, G. (2006). *Indigenous peoples and diabetes: Community empowerment and wellness.* Durham: Carolina Academic Press.

Gholap, N., Davies, M., Patel, K., Sattar, N., & Khunti, K. (2011). Type 2 diabetes and cardiovascular disease in South Asians. *Primary Care Diabetes, 5,* 45–56.

Giddens, A. (1991). *Modernity and self-identity.* Cambridge: Polity Press.

Gilroy, P. (2012). My Britain is fuck all' zombie multiculturalism and the race politics of citizenship. *Identities: Global Studies in Culture and Power, 19*(4), 380–397.

Happe, K. (2013). *The material gene: Gender, race and heredity after the human genome project.* New York: New York University Press.

Hedgecoe, A. (2001). Ethical boundary work: Geneticization, philosophy and the social sciences. *Medicine Health Care and Philosophy, 4,* 305–309.

Hedgecoe, A. (2002). Reinventing diabetes: Classification, division and the geneticization of a disease. *New Genetics and Society, 21*(1), 7–27.

Hill, C. (1969). *Immigration and integration.* Devon: Perganon Press.

Hiro, D. (1992). *Black British, White British.* London: Grafton Books.

Hex, N., Bartlett, C., Wright, D., Taylor, M., & Varley, D. (2012). Estimating the current and future costs of Type 1 and Type 2 diabetes in the UK, including direct health costs and indirect societal and productivity costs. *Diabetic Medicine, 29*(7), 855–862. doi: 10.1111/j.1464-5491.2012.03698.x.

International Diabetes Federation. (2013). *IDF diabetes atlas* (6th ed.). Brussels: International Diabetes Federation. Available at: http://idf.org/diabetesatlas/download-book. Accessed 2 Jul 2014.

Krieger, N. (2001). Theories for social epidemiology in the 21st Century: An eco-social approach. *International Journal of Epidemiology, 30*(4), 668–677.

Lambert, H., & Sevak, M. (1996). Is cultural difference a useful concept? Perceptions of health and sources of ill health among Londoners of South Asian origin. In D. Kelleher & S. Hillier (Eds.), *Researching cultural differences in health*. London: Routledge.

Lawton, J. (2003). Lay experiences of health and illness: Past research and future agendas. *Sociology of Health and Illness, 25*, 23–40.

McKeigue, P. M., & Marmot, M. G. (1988). Mortality from coronary heart disease in Asian communities in London. *British Medical Journal, 297*, 903.

McKeigue, P., Miller, G. J., & Marmot, M. G. (1989). Coronary heart disease in South Asians overseas – A review. *Journal of Clinical Epidemiology, 42*, 597–609.

Mendenhall, E., Seligman, R., Fernandez, A., & Jacobs, E. (2010). Speaking through diabetes: Rethinking the significance of lay discourses on diabetes. *Medical Anthropology Quarterly, 24*(2), 220–239. ISSN 0745-5194, online ISSN 1548-1387.

Mokdad, A. H., Bowman, B. A., Ford, E. S., Vinicor, F., Marks, J. S., & Koplan, J. P. (2001). The continuing epidemics of obesity and diabetes in the United States. *Journal of the American Medical Association, 286*, 1195–1200.

Montoya, M. J. (2011). *Making the Mexican diabetic: Race, science, and the genetics of inequality*. London: University of California Press.

Mooy, J. M., de Vries, H., Grootenhuis, P. A., Bouter, L. M., & Heine, R. J. (2000). Major stressful life events in relation to prevalence of undetected type 2 diabetes: The Hoorn Study. *Diabetes Care, 23*(2), 197–201.

Nagi, D. (2004). Diabetes: A challenge for health professionals and policy makers. In S. Ali & K. Atkin (Eds.), *Primary healthcare and South Asian populations* (pp. 89–100). Oxon: Radcliffe Medical Press.

Nazroo, J. Y. (2003). The structuring of ethnic inequalities in health: Economic position, racial discrimination, and racism. *American Journal of Public Health, 93*(2), 277–284. Available at: http://ajph.aphapublications.org/doi/abs/10.2105/AJPH.93.2.277.

Oldroyd, J., Banerjee, M., Heald, A., & Cruickshank, K. (2005). Diabetes and ethnic minorities. *Postgraduate Medical Journal, 81*, 486–490. doi:10.1136/pgmj.2004.029124.

Popay, J., Williams, G., Thomas, C., & Gatrell, T. (1998). Theorising inequalities in health: The place of lay knowledge. *Sociology of Health & Illness, 20*(5), 619–644.

Prior, L. (2003). Belief, knowledge and expertise: The emergence of the lay expert in medical sociology. *Sociology of Health & Illness, 25*(Silver Anniversary Issue), 41–57.

Radley, A., & Billig, M. (1996). Accounts of health and illness: Dilemmas and representations. *Sociology of Health & Illness, 18*(2), 220–240.

Rajaram, S. S. (1997). Experience of hypoglycaemia among insulin dependent diabetics and its impact on the family. *Sociology of Health and Illness, 19*(3), 281–296.

Rock, M. (2003). Sweet blood and social suffering: Rethinking cause–effect relationships in diabetes, distress and duress. *Medical Anthropology, 22,* 131–174.

Rubin, A. L. (2001). *Diabetes for dummies.* New York: Wiley.

Scheper-Hughes, N. (2006). Diabetes and genocide-beyond the thrifty gene. In M. Ferreira & G. Lang (Eds.), *Indigenous peoples and diabetes: Community empowerment and wellness.* Durham: Carolina Academic Press.

Simmons, D., Williams, D. R., & Powell, M. J. (1992). Prevalence of diabetes in different regional and religious South Asian communities in Coventry. *Diabetic Medicine, 9*(5), 428–431.

Subbulakshmi, G., & Naik, M. (2001). Indigenous foods in the treatment of diabetes mellitus. *Bombay Hospital Journal, 43,* 4.

Turner, S. (2001). What's the problem with experts? *Social Studies of Science, 31*(1), 123–149.

UKPDS. (1998). Ethnicity and cardiovascular disease. The incidence of myocardial infarction in White, South Asian, and Afro-Caribbean patients with type 2 diabetes (U.K. Prospective Diabetes Study 32). *Diabetes-Care, 21*(8), 1271–1277.

Visram, R. (2002). *Asians in Britain: 400 years of history.* London: Pluto.

Wild, S., & Chaturvedi, N. (2009). Epidemiology. In K. Khunti & S. Kumar (Eds.), *Diabetes UK and South Asian Health Foundation recommendations on Diabetes research priorities for British South Asians* (1st ed., pp. 12–20). London: Diabetes UK.

Wild, S., & Forouhi, N. (2009). Epidemiology. In K. Khunti, S. Kumar, & J. Brodie (Eds.), *Diabetes UK and South Asian Health Foundation recommendations on diabetes research priorities for British South Asians.* London: Diabetes UK.

Williams, G. (1984). The genesis of chronic illness: Narrative reconstruction. *Sociology of Health and Illness, 6*(2), 175–200.

World Health Organization. (2013). World Diabetes Day 2012. www.who.int/diabetes/en

4

Constructing the Risk: Faulty Lifestyles, Faulty Genes

Within the debate concerning diabetes prevalence and ethnicity, there are a number of well-documented lines along which the arguments progress. 'Lifestyle' factors such as diet and exercise are regularly proposed as important elements of the argument, especially when linked to ideas surrounding the 'acculturation' process. In this chapter, I highlight the ways in which the 'risky' South Asian diabetic body—and the discourses that surround, and therefore, generate its material reality—utilise notions of fault, culpability, and individual responsibility. These are manifested in a number of ways, from the content and manner of food consumption, to the alleged inability or unwillingness to conform to societal health norms regarding normalised health protection practices. The fault lines also extend to the somewhat troubling notion of genetic science, and the genetic predisposition thesis, which has been long applied to the study of diabetes.

Dietary forms in societies in the West are often said to be characterised by lowered fibre, increased animal fats, and processed foods, and these have been associated with a higher predisposition to diabetes, through higher obesity levels (Hu 2011). Consumption of fats and refined carbohydrates are also factors in increased predisposition to obesity and type 2 diabetes—the risk of diabetes increases by 4.5 times for every 1 kg of

© The Editor(s) (if applicable) and The Author(s) 2016
H. Keval, *Health, Ethnicity and Diabetes*,
DOI 10.1057/978-1-137-45703-5_4

weight gain. This, in turn, is related to reduced levels of physical activity, also associated with the 'Westernisation' hypothesis (Manson et al. 1991).

Studies in the USA have consistently shown that the diets of migrants have, over time and generations, changed to include more fat, sodium, sugar, and calories. The global diabetes epidemic and the specific centres of prevalence—which, according to the International Diabetes Federation, (IDF) are China and India—are driven by 'rapid urbanisation, nutrition transition and increasingly sedentary lifestyles' (Hu 2011: 1255). Gupta et al.'s study (1995) implied that South Asians could be seen as a genetically distinct group—a race—who used too much 'ghee' (clarified butter) for cooking and experienced a consistent lack of exercise—all of which have been refuted by other theorists (Abate and Chandalia 2003). Furthermore, researchers such as Hill (2006) reproblematise South Asian 'cultures' by making generalised claims about South Asian diets lacking in fruit and vegetables, and lifestyles lacking in exercise. While alerting us to the need for sensitive and specific diabetes healthcare, this seems to invoke the 'cultural pathology' notions of the past. The epidemiology of diabetes is not in question, but placing the burden of responsibility on '...aspects of South Asian culture' (Hill 2006: 64) needs to be considered with caution, as this offers little of theoretical or practical value, and increases the prevalence of stereotypes and caricatures. The explanatory utility of these various approaches is questionable, not least because it may well be conceptually and empirically rather difficult to define what precisely a homogenous 'South Asian culture' is.

Research which examines the interaction of 'ethnicity' and diet does not seem to produce a strong argument. Schonfield et al.'s (1987) study comparing Asian Indian men and European men—both vegetarian—showed the Indians in this study as having increased insulin resistance, despite having identical nutritional intake, yet other studies have shown that diet alone did not contribute to insulin resistance (Sevak et al. 1994). When one considers the traditional diet of many people within South Asian groups (especially Hindu Gujaratis)—vegetables, pulses, and rice—it is difficult to imagine the 'dietary composition' argument holding any ground as an explanatory factor for high diabetes levels. In fact, as McKeigue et al. (1989) and Matheson et al. (1985) demonstrate, aspects of the South Asian diet actually form a protection against some conditions, such as colo-rectal cancer. The misinformation regarding the generalised supposed unhealthy diet may well be a historical remnant of the health campaigns for the increased rickets syndrome in the South Asian community during the last three decades (Rocheron 1988) or the incorrect assumption in research and health education materials that general fat content is too high in these diets (Bhatt and Dickinson 1992; Silman et al. 1985).

Exercise and activity have also been at the forefront of both explanations and interventions for diabetes sufferers. The health intervention aspects of promoting exercise and activity for people with the disease are based on medical and biological evidence (Ramachandran et al. 2013; NICE 2012b, c), all of which demonstrate that exercise functions to control weight and improve insulin resistance. However, the ideas linked to various ethnic groupings lacking activity and exercise are unproblematised and foster a culture of blame rather than sensitive and appropriate healthcare—much like the 'culturalist' explanations utilised in the late 1980s and early 1990s, shown to be flawed, and which 'pathologised' (Ahmad 1993) minority health issues. Although sedentary lifestyles have been associated with generalised obesity in urban environments, McKeigue et al. (1992) show that, actually, it is not the lack of activity in general, or work activity, but the lack of leisure time activity, which showed a decrease (associated with health and fitness activity programmes) among Asian Indians in the UK. This seems to echo Ahmad's (1993) vehement argument against pathologising 'culture' and 'ethnicity', and seeking a more socio-politically based explanation, which would account for inequalities in health status based on socio-economic positions. The notion of 'lifestyle', which, in most popular health discourse, includes a whole range of entities, including diet and exercise, is an invention borne of particular time periods and processes within Western European development. O'Brien's (1995) discussion of the origins of 'lifestyle' is of particular relevance here, because the direction which health discourse has taken over the last three decades has demonstrably utilised late modern notions of personal and individual choice and responsibility. O'Brien refers to Weberian frameworks, which focused on social status, Simmel's work on the philosophy of money, and Adler's use of the term 'lifestyle' to explore personalised expressions in increasingly complicated social worlds (O'Brien 1995). For these authors who were writing, reacting to, and investigating the rapid modernisation of everyday personal, social, and cultural life, lifestyle was an idea to be used to explore how social actors navigated the turbulence and continuity of increasingly complex political, economic, and cultural contexts. We can see that these early ideas of lifestyle have been transformed in line with the political landscape over the last three decades of health discourse.

As O'Brien states,

> ...lifestyle...has emerged as a vehicle for differentiating populations, for breaking it apart, fragmenting its interests and distancing its members from forms of collective, social action...embodying a moment of political change...the association between 'health' and 'lifestyle' is fundamentally a political achievement, supported by an institutionalised consumerism, validated by a liberal political ideology and nurtured by a technocratic pro-fessionalism increasingly oriented towards problem solving approaches to health and social life. (1995: 193)

In many ways, this speaks to one of the central concerns of this book: that the picture of South Asian health—diabetes in particular—has gradually been rendered as a 'problem' for both public and private health to solve. The continuous provision of scientific, epidemiological, and 'lifestyle' remedies presume the existence of faulty cultures and faulty genes.

The intersection of three focal elements in this discussion contributes to our understanding of this particular part of the picture: first, rigorous diabetes science and epidemiology, which we can translate as counting various units of measurement *within* the body; second, health promo-tion, in a sense, counting the socially and materially mediated spaces *between* bodies; and finally, lifestyle (including diets), which can be viewed as counting and evaluating acts of normative compliance *using* the body. When combined, these result in a discursive formation (Foucault 1972), resulting in a construction of risk, which ultimately presents itself as benign, just, and an integral part of the dissemination of health information, and provision of services. In a sense, this imposes a normative order on unruly, ethno-cultural specific bodies that have become the special focus of a particular gaze.

Linking the Personal and the Public: Diabetes as 'Trouble' and 'Issue'

The presence of scientific information regarding the efficacy of 'healthy eating', the positive impacts of regular exercise, and an 'appropriate' use of healthcare provision, all presume that the fundamental causes of the increased risk can be mitigated by 'lifestyle' changes—hence, the consistent and powerful recommendations by NICE to medical practitioners for advising intensive lifestyle changes to anyone within the high risk group (NICE 2012a, b, c). While the dissemination of such protective recommendations regarding such risk screening might be seen as essential in light of the differential prevalence and incidence rates so often repeated, the coalface impact is less than straightforward. I illustrate this with an example from my own experiences, an academic writing practice which utilises, in this brief example, the auto/biographical approach (Murji 2008). When I present myself to my GP surgery, I appear as a mid-40s male, British South Asian in origin. The advice I am automatically given, regardless of any personal, socio-economic, material, biographical, or socio-cultural context, is that I am at a higher risk of acquiring diabetes than another mid-40s male, with an identical profile, who happens to be classified as 'White'. There are a number of problems with this, not least the fact that the entire basis on which I am categorised using the label 'South Asian high risk' is a flawed, pseudo-scientific enterprise. I am African by birth, Indian and Burmese by parental origin, British by citizenship, BrAsian (Ali et al. 2006) by contemporary postcolonial, social, and cultural identity. I also variously, selectively, identify according to differential consumption patterns and lifestyles, and yet, my 'risk' category is generated on the basis of a series of raciological labels derived by a scientific enterprise that relies on spurious associations between vague notions of 'race', 'ethnic' origin, and a geopolitical category (South Asian). In the UK, between the 1991 and 2011 census, the number of 'identity' tick boxes grew from 9 to 18, and yet, the most recent list of categories still does not contain any categories for African Asians, nor, as Murji (2008) found, an 'East African Asian' category, despite the presence of African Asians in the UK for many years, even prior to the infamous

Ugandan expulsion in 1972. This is despite the fact of a distinct East African Asian migration pattern since the 1960s (Brah 2006).

When my partner, prior to the birth of our second child, visited the health centre for a routine check-up, as is 'normal' practice, one of the first striking comments we were presented with was that as we were 'Asian', and therefore, a 'high diabetes risk', we should undergo extra tests in order to make sure that she was screened appropriately. I concede this is anecdotal, personalised, and therefore, 'unscientific' in many ways. But, in the tradition of Mills (1959), I use this 'personal trouble' and explore how it can potentially be revealed as a 'public issue'. Indeed, if we look at the NICE guidelines and advice to practitioners nationwide, then clearly, healthcare providers are carrying out the instructions as provided by an official government body—making this very much a public issue. The problem lies in several steps before this ultimate face-to-face encounter. The conceptualisation of difference, the use of these categories in research and intervention, and the alignment of flawed notions of 'cultural' pathology, which endure in both research and practice, culminate in a very particular practice that is qualitatively and experientially different to a comparative counterpart who was categorised as 'White', for example. My anecdote indicates that at the coal-face encounter, what is being utilised is a subtle combination of 'scientific' evidence about prevalence and incidence, the as-yet-to-be-supported 'genetic predisposition' to risks thesis, and 'risky' inappropriate lifestyle habits. Taken in combination, this 'risk package' performs a metonymic function. In other words, the moment a tick box is checked to indicate a specific 'ethnic' category, specific racialised risk constructions come into play.

The label 'South Asian' within diabetes discourse has taken on the burden of carrying a huge and problematic risk baggage—a burden which is also transferred to people who inadvertently fall into this grouping. As Karlsen and Laia (2012) have shown, even where lifestyle is empirically interpreted and mobilised in research as health-related behaviour, there is great variation within as well as between ethnic groups, and in addition, any differences in lifestyles cannot in themselves explain the inequalities between them. Attempting to pinpoint a nebulous and vague sociopolitical late modern health construct and using it to frame causes *and* to effect health change needs to be thought through very carefully, in light of the overwhelming impact of socio-economic disadvantage and racialised victimisation (Nazroo and Karlsen 2002). These 'lifestyle' arguments are mobilised in ethno-diabetes discourse as both explanations and remedies for cultural pathologies, essentially speaking to the racialisation of cultural difference. The evidence, as Karlsen and Laia (2012) argue, directs us to wider possibilities, such as the way in which institutionalised cultures of healthcare provision may perpetuate disadvantages. The argument for critical authors is strongly in favour of the complex interplay of structural and socio-economic disadvantage, migration, and the enduring legacies of racism, but we can also identify that the neo-liberal, health promotion, 'lifestyle' direction of health policies in recent years may have had many multifactorial effects on the topic of 'ethno-diabetes'.

The Politics of 'Ethnic' Diabetes

Without any doubt, the physiological reality of diabetes necessitates health policy approaches to mitigate the impacts on the national health burden. As the rates of the disease increase across the globe and nationally, the economic costs often figure prominently in the discourse. It is not within the scope of this book to critically analyse the entirety of government policy in relation to diabetes and ethnicity, but for the purpose of excavating further nuances in the risk construction process, some forays into policy will serve the function. Health policy is not a single, neutral position, but rather, a range of normative, economically and ideologically contrived prescriptions that, at once, both give the appearance of *reacting to* epidemiological data, indicating focused health needs, and pro-actively shaping the health patterns via a number of behavioural and economic models. By this, I mean that in the traditional sociological sense, there is always a strong ideological focus in health policy, which implicitly positions itself in a range of foci. These are quite explicitly related to the notion of responsibility over one's health. The movement in late modernity of health concerns towards health promotion is underwritten by patterns of contemporary consumer society (Bunton and Burrows 1995). With health being underpinned by individual responsibility and a shift away from traditional hospital-centred medicine towards the promotion of particular lifestyles, how health agencies then react to and work within this shifting paradigm is interesting. This different way of conceptualising health involves the notion of 'health roles' (Bunton and Burrows 1995: 208). This can be observed in the way that diabetes prevention and management becomes more aligned to the extent to which *individuals change their lifestyles*. During the years after the NHS was established and successive governments attempted to handle the unpredictable and overwhelming demand on the health service (Ham et al. 2012), the political ideologies underwriting the healthcare system within the UK were clearly visible. As Bloch et al. point out, 'health research, policymaking, service delivery and practice can be understood as evolving in relation to the increasingly complex compositions of multiculture' (2013: 128). This raises questions for our discussion of policy approaches to diabetes and ethnicity. If the way in which health is conceptualised, researched, and acted upon by policy makers is shaped by corresponding ideations of race relations, then surely, policies which deal with a manifestly 'ethnic' high risk potential, such as diabetes, might also reflect these patterns of thinking?

As governments attempt to structure the health service in terms of financially viable approaches to public health (Ham 2009)—a concern which quickly became an emergent issue with the popularity of the NHS in its early years—they also work within specific paradigms of health. As the NHS has developed over the last 60 years, it has needed to adapt to changes in government, changing health profiles in the populations, demographic changes, and global financial contexts. In addition to this, as governments come and go, each political formulation of health heralds a different organisational ethos and structure, with corresponding funding arrangements These arrangements and reorganisations all have an impact on how health is thought about and experienced—both at the patient/service user level and at the service provider level (see Ham 2009). By far, the biggest change to the NHS arrived as a result of the conservative government of Margaret Thatcher in 1979. There is fair consensus that the UK healthcare system has never really recovered from the introduction of internal markets ('quasi-markets'), and what has been termed the 'neo-liberalisation' of healthcare (McGregor 2001). Certainly, the current pressure placed on the NHS is part of the overall historical, and continuing political, context within which this structure sits. Estimates place the required financial spending on the NHS at £8 billion per year by 2020 if a crisis is to be avoided (Kings Fund 2015). The prevailing winds of American political change in the late 1970s and beyond left a more right-of-centre, conservative sense of individualism in its wake, and UK political scenery changed in light of this in the 1980s. So too, there was a corresponding change in how the government dealt with, or managed, 'difference'. Ahmad and Bradby (2007) explain the early 'health politics' reaction to post-war migrants was riddled with problematic and narrowly conceptualised notions of difference, leading to 'ethnic-specific' policy of health campaigns. These 'ethnic-specific' health and welfare services, therefore, were developed at both national and localised levels, and reflected what Ahmad and Bradby (2007) and others call 'crude multiculturalism', 'which stripped minority cultures of their complexity, contingency and dynamism' (2007: 804). Added to this, of course, is the 'delicious irony' (Kyriakides and Virdee (2003: 287) of migrant labour having to be contracted into the UK from the Commonwealth to build the NHS and welfare state system during expansion as emblematic of the power of Empire, and which could only be achieved by calling on colonial subjects who had been historically viewed as inferior subjects.

The dialectical process of power relations between groups within this given polity resulted in a corresponding reaction, in what was labelled 'anti-racism'—a mainly activist but also academic-inspired movement which acknowledged and combatted deeply embedded racialised inequality in British society. For this to be effective, there needed to be a unifying of the hitherto differentiated ethnic categories imposed by policies, so that a 'Black' unity would emerge, mobilising resistance at all levels of societal racial injustice. Anti-racist resistance movements came across an unfaltering Conservative government stance on immigration, race, and ethnic minority management (Farrar 2004), but continued to challenge hegemonic stances on race relations in Britain. As Flynn and Craig (2012) indicate, new forms of 'race' questions emerged, as pluralities and hybridities in identities were identified in the 'new multiculturalism'. Forms of cultural difference could sit alongside acknowledgement and analysis of structural disadvantage, so the scene was set for a potentially rich sociopolitical formulation of difference. Unfortunately, as the late 1990s and

2000s demonstrated, changes in government and political attitudes to immigration and settled BME communities in the UK led to discourses of 'Britishness'. The fundamental issue was the perception that migrants had brought with them specific cultural ways and values. The overwhelming critique then, and currently, is that if people retain these cultural values, there will be groups of people with what many UK political parties have called 'British values' and minority groups who will fail to absorb and learn these prescriptive, mythical notions of 'British values' (critiqued extensively, e.g. Keval 2014; Lentin and Titley 2011). Such clashes lead to communities purpotedly self-segregating over several generations (see Cantle 2012), and therefore, demonstrate what many have called the failure or (contested) 'death' of multiculturalism (Pitcher 2009; Farrar et al. 2012). The current manifestation of government policy on dealing with 'difference' is not very far from the original assimilationist policies of the 1960s (Flynn and Craig 2012). I do not wish to rehearse a fully developed account of multiculturalism and its associated debates, summaries of which can be found in Lentin and Titley (2011), Bloch et al. (2013), and Pitcher (2009). As the political backdrop to 'dealing with difference' changes and accommodates official policy formulations, so too do health policies and how they conceptualise the health of the nation's minority populations. The lens through which researchers, policy makers, academics, and service provides view people of different ethnicities, languages, religions, and cultures will, in turn, construct a specific racialised gaze.

Regardless of where political affiliations lie, it is clear that the politics of health has an impact on how health policies are formulated, and crucially, for diabetes, how the experiences of minorities are to be dealt with. Such connections are apparent in how the government, over the last 20 years or so, has engaged with 'minority' health, discussions about migrants, immigration, race and racism, and colonial legacies. As the UK government has, decade after decade, attempted to 'manage race relations' (Flynn and Craig 2012), there has been a corresponding effect on concepts of health and health services. The original, liberal-oriented welfare state of Aneurin Bevan evolved—some would say 'eroded'—so the notion of 'responsibility' for one's own health became a prime focus for governments to encourage. I have already discussed the ways in which specific conditions were attached by policy makers and researchers to specific ethnic groups, resulting in pathologisation of communities, effectively racialising health. These are examples of how difficult UK health policy makers find the process of embedding equality into the healthcare services. Flynn and Craig's (2012) discussion of the way in which 'race' relations was 'managed' from the 1960s to current events reflects the various changes in political treatments of migration and race, from assimilation to multiculturalism, to community cohesion. Each of these broad eras contains details of precisely how racially, culturally, and ethnically defined groups 'fitted' into British society and the according response from the government. Health policy too takes on the hues and shades of political attitudes to difference.

Ethnicity-Related Diabetes Initiatives

While many of the arguments and observations I make are of a historical nature, mainly related to the management of difference since post-war immigration, there are more recent examples of health policy work, which indicate the difficulties some government bodies experience in thinking through ethnicity and health. In a research review from 2002, the Department of Health and the Medical Research Council attempted to address the rise in diabetes cases in minority communities. The recommended method was implementation of 'Innovative lifestyle educational methods', which 'involve working with Indian restaurants to provide low fat alternatives on their menus' (2002: 129). Although these fat-reducing and calorie-lowering techniques are popular in much of what I call the health-nutrition industry discourse, many of these research and practice initiatives consistently ignore the multilayered and complex web of social and material contexts in which calorie consumption takes place. Reducing the amount of unhealthy fats consumed by people may well have physiological and public health logic behind it, but the theoretical and practical nature of specific minority group targeting needs to be questioned. Such a 're-imagining (of) the social in the nutrition sciences' (Schubert et al. 2012: 352) not only requires us to view the 'social' as contributory, but rather is central to our concerns, especially in relation to socio-economic status.

The impact of health campaigns and welfare agencies which target groups identified by a marker of difference based on unpacked concepts may range from immediate concrete stereotypes influencing healthcare provision, to long-term systemic and institutional issues (see Patel 1993; Johnson 1993; Salway et al. 2007, 2013). One would need to question the value of using low-fat menus in Indian restaurants to combat the diabetes issue in South Asian communities, with specific reference to the target audience. The question needs to be asked: is there a group of South Asian mature onset diabetes sufferers who regularly visit Indian restaurants, and if so, would having a low-fat menu make a difference to the overall incidence and prevalence rates? If indeed there is empirical evidence which indicates that: (1) South Asian people in the UK who are at high risk of diabetes are more likely to frequent 'Indian' restaurants than other groups, and (2) this visiting of 'Indian' restaurants is empirically proven to be a contributory factor in the diabetes rates, then perhaps, we might look upon such initiatives as potentially a useful segment in the overall race-health equality picture. There is also the additional question of whether or not all the other ethnic groups, who may also have a likelihood of suffering from particular conditions related to obesity, coronary heart disease, and diabetes, also have 'their' eating establishments equipped with low-fat menus. There is a broader issue of the label 'Indian restaurants', given the view that this is not a homogenous group and is as internally disparate and distinct as the term 'South Asian'. It is unclear how this strategy might impact the experience of diabetes management and health maintenance of South Asian type 2 diabetics. Embedded within this line of reasoning is the assumption that there is something 'faulty' within the 'South Asian diet which requires a 'fix' of some sort, reverting health analysis to the older models of 'cultural pathology'. Though health promotion has been under the watchful critique of sociology (Bunton et al. 1995), as has health promotion for ethnic minorities (Bhopal and White 1993), there is a persistent production of discourse which reinforces simplistic notions of minority culture, and of what that minority or 'other' identity entails.

Related to this policy-level action is the work of organisations which manage and coordinate support networks for people with diabetes. Diabetes UK is a national network for advice, support, information, and health promotion activities. It has gained a prominent position in the field, both in terms of its engagement with the lives of people who have diabetes and as a conduit for biomedical research, and provides multilingual information to a number of BME groups. The intensive and extensive contributions to people's lives notwithstanding, it is interesting for us to explore how organisations involved in the health management of diabetes are also responsible for discourses in knowledge production.

In a 2003 online publication which provided guidance on 'cultural sensitivity', we are told that

> Hindus and Sikhs believe in reincarnation—as a result, many believe that their suffering from health-related causes is 'paying for sins that may have taken place in their previous life'. Many refuse to take medication because they see health conditions as 'an act of God' that is written in their destiny. Similarly many people from the Afro-Caribbean communities are highly superstitious and see 'having health conditions as a curse' (Diabetes UK 2003)

Regardless of the intention here—which ostensibly is to provide some form of information about the diversity in people's belief systems which may impact on their health, the impact on health providers and clients is potentially problematic. BME communities, here doubled up as ethno-religious faith communities, are constructed as somehow basic in their abilities to negotiate complex social, physical, and emotional landscapes. Through homogenising internally diverse groups, they are rendered passive and helpless due to supposed strict religion, faith, or superstition. Clearly, there is room for a more sophisticated approach, and this academic/intervention impact space has fortunately recently been occupied by more nuanced and considered approaches (e.g. Stone et al. 2005, 2013). As the book aims to show in later chapters, the relationship between cultural/ethnic identity and religion/faith and health is far more nuanced and complex than may be reflected in prevailing 'fatalism' narratives.

Of course, the questions that are not being asked or addressed in ethno-religious veiling of this type is how these 'cultural' formulations of non-compliance are any different to any other types of non-compliance enacted by other groups? For example, Oldroyd et al. (2005) in their review of the relationship between ethnicity and diabetes establish a correlational and descriptive link between diabetes prevalence and ethnic groups. Although this correlation is presented as epidemiologically neutral, they go on to infer that while GP consultations were more frequent in African-Caribbean communities, for Pakistani and Indian groups (findings generally corroborated by research), 'barriers to care include poor understanding of the severity of symptoms, poor communication, knowledge of the value of preventative care, knowledge about the availability of services' (2005: 489) whilst citing research indicating that *'South Asians have been found to be less likely to be given follow up GP appointments…to be offered district nurse services…and have had previous cardiological consultation'* (2005: 489). The discursive function of this form of 'scientific' representation is to focus on (and misunderstand) descriptive correlations between variables, and gloss over the vital, contextual underpinnings of health inequality-related patterns. As Ricci-Cabello et al. (2010) confirmed in their meta-analysis of studies focusing on diabetes prevention and inequalities, even in countries which are economically developed and with universal healthcare systems in place, there still exists the enduring intersection of ethnicity and socio-economic inequalities. Structural and material constellations of disadvantage, which themselves are generated and perpetuated by cycles of racialised inequality, have a pivotal role to play in minority health status and experience.

Guidelines for both practitioners and the lay public, as demonstrated in a variety of NICE policies, are keen to prioritise the achievement of equality, especially since the 2010 Equality Act, which synergised a variety of 'protected characteristics', such as race, age, gender, disability, and sexuality, and faith under one legal, enforceable protective framework. As public bodies are keen to address the potential issues involved in serving a multicultural society, organisations which deliver healthcare, in the UK NHS (though the system itself is characterised by multiple fragmentations in its governance, management, hierarchy, and accountability; see Ham 2009 for more discussion on this) have also seen shifts in the preponderance of 'cultural sensitivity' components. While many such movements in healthcare delivery are warranted—or example, translation services—other patterns are more subtle. For example, in 2012, NICE published guidance on the prevention of diabetes at the population level.

A part of this was directed at higher risks groups: 'those aged 25–39 and of South Asian, Chinese, African-Caribbean or Black African descent, and other high risk and minority ethnic (BME)' (NICE 2012a). The recommendations focus on two activities: (1) identifying people at risk, which involves a risk assessment score and a blood test, and (2) providing lifestyle change programmes. Both of these activities are supported by a plethora of scientific knowledge bases. However, from a critical sociological perspective, perhaps echoing Montoya (2011) and others (Bliss 2011; Rock 2005), we can see that both of these are examples of the same discursive constructions that have been discussed earlier in this book. The process of risk identification assumes and preconceives in a positivist fashion, that categories of 'high risk' are freely available, value- and ideology-free, fixed and attached to categories of people, existing in the embodied minority population, awaiting collection by and for scientific reporting. In this series of expert diabetes narratives, corroborated and validated by the prevailing system of knowledge production, Castel's (1991, cited in Bunton and Burrows 1995: 209) subject clinic becomes translated into the epidemiology clinic, in which 'systematic pre-detection' facilitates the categorisation, indexing, labelling, and management of populations. BME populations which have long been the object of scrutiny and 'diversity management' become, in epidemiological terms, part of the 'risk package' to be managed.

The second part of the NICE activities is driven by the discourse of cultural deficit. By enforcing strategies of lifestyle change, there can be very little space to challenge the legitimated authority, which defines, organises, and ratifies normative cultural prescriptions of 'lifestyle'. The extensive plethora of information guidelines, held within the NICE platform is organised under 'pathways', guidance, standards, indicators, evidence, and services (see http://www.nice.org.uk). It is disseminated to health professionals in reassuringly comprehensive 'scientific' coverage, but dizzyingly cavernous in its range. Whilst aligning itself with the contemporary Equalities Act-driven agenda, and mobilising multiple resources to work within 'cultural sensitivity', the majority of the knowledge base on diabetes and ethnicity revolves around several main notions. First, that people categorised as 'South Asian' (bearing in mind my comments earlier about the problematic use of this category) ARE at higher risk of getting diabetes, experiencing related complications, presenting to and accessing the healthcare system later; second, this group (South Asians) IS at higher risk of truncal obesity (accumulation of fat around the stomach), which places extra pressure on the cardiovascular system and functions as a risk indicator of diabetes and coronary heart disease; and finally, South Asians between specific ages ARE to be risk assessed, and then, appropriately placed within lifestyle intervention change programmes. The connection between truncal obesity and a range of cardiovascular and diabetes-related problems has now found firm purchase within the South Asian risk category, demonstrated both in NICE guidelines (NICE 2012) as well as in research (see, e.g., Bhopal 2013; Khunti et al. 2009; McKeigue et al. 1991, 1992; Misra et al. 2009). The NHS choices website, a service user-oriented site with information, guidance, and support for the public contains a 'South Asian Health Issues' section, which warns of the increased body mass index (BMI) problem for South Asians. In clear terms, useful for non-medical experts, it warns people that a BMI score of 23 or more results in an increased risk, while 27.5 represents a high risk ('South Asian' people are subject to a different BMI cut-off point for high risk than 'White' people). This information is prefaced by a narrative now familiar in both academic scientific as well as lay discourse—namely, the 'risk package'. This documents the basic statistical multipliers in prevalence and incidence, followed by the routine explanatory disclaimers regarding uncertainty about the causes. The uncertainty about the cause of these increased risks is immediately followed by the diet, lifestyle, and evolutionary fat storage narratives, in a sense, negating the bio-physiological uncertainty by juxtaposing it with the 'cultural deficit' certainty. This peculiar and tensioned relation is not rare—Renee Fox (1980, 2007), amongst others (Atkinson 1984), has explored the idea of medical and health-related certainty and uncertainty in some detail. In this case, it relates to the kind of picture which is rendered when our critical gaze ceases to limit its focus on individual and group risk statistics, and begins to observe wider patterns of knowledge production, and the forces and impacts involved in this production. As I have already mentioned, the 'risk package'—a set of discourses—are here being presented as de facto and incontestable truths, when, in reality, there is a whole range of conceptual and theoretical complexities inherent in the relationship between a racialised, geopolitical category such as 'South Asian', and the notion of 'risk'. As I argue above, there are multiple sites of constructing the 'South Asian risky body', and culture, lifestyle, and as discussed below, genetics become some of the principle ways in which these constructions are revealed as racialised and problematic.

The 'Thrifty Gene': Genetic Arguments, Diabetes, and Ethnicity

As a powerful correlate in studies of cardiovascular diseases and diabetes in general, obesity is often used as a catch-all explanatory term, resulting in a new term that has been introduced into the literature—'diabesity' (Shafrir 1996; McNaughton 2013). Biologically, obesity has been linked to the development of insulin resistance. The development of type 2 diabetes begins with glucose tolerance impairment, which gradually develops into the 'metabolic syndrome', a cluster of risk factors, of which one of the most important is obesity (Zimmett and Thomas 2003). Other writers, such as Abate and Chandalia (2003) and Zimmett and Thomas (2003), argue for a primary metabolic defect—a genetic predisposition which, when interacting with the environment, causes a much higher type 2 diabetes prevalence rate. However, more recent arguments surrounding this issue with relevance to ethnicity and in particular South Asians address the way in which fat is distributed around the body. Abdominal, truncal, or central obesity, has been shown in higher number of certain ethnic groups than others (Gilbert et al. 1992; Hu et al. 2001). Asian Indians reportedly have higher waist to hip ratios and thicker skin folds compared to Europeans with comparable BMIs (Mckeigue et al. 1991). As Hu (2011) and Yajnik (2001), amongst many others, argue, South Asians as revealed in the epidemiology show a tendency to carry more fat around central or truncal regions. However, this is seen as a contributory factor rather than a single explanatory mechanism. One of the problematic tendencies is to over extend the biological/epidemiological/physiological science to areas where all-encompassing explanations are generated. Indeed, Abate and Chandalia (2001) showed that in a controlled trial, when compared with Caucasians, neither obesity nor fat distribution could explain high insulin resistance and type 2 diabetes. The complexity of the combination of factors within South Asian diabetes is somewhat simplified and made more convenient by the metonymic tendency of diabetes risk discourse. The general 'risk package' here is perpetuated in terms of the presentation of urbanisation and Westernisation, availability of food and the related idea of 'over-nutrition' and 'under-nutrition' (Hu 2011), truncal obesity, and development of diabetes at a lower BMI (Yajnik 2001; Hu 2011; Bhopal 2013). This is compounded by the combination of foetal under nutrition and Westernised lifestyles and diets in later life (Hales and Barker 2001). This combination of factors is now the accepted route to scientific legitimacy within diabetes discourses around South Asian groups, but the final factor—intrauterine environments adapting to or reacting to external environments—leads inexorably to the possibility of what Bhopal (2013) in his four-stage model called a 'small, relatively fatty baby' (2013: 36). While the scientific evidence for this consists of a now established empirical trail, this discussion of obesity ultimately leads to the scientific logical next step— genetic arguments. Whilst I provide a more detailed discussion of the problematic relationship between race, diabetes, and genetic predispositions elsewhere (see Keval 2015), here, I summarise some key ideas in order to complement the overall picture of constructing a South Asian diabetes risk.

Genetic mutations of insulin receptors have been reported, although they are known to be infrequently occurring. The 'thrifty gene' hypothesis (Neel 1962, cited in Ferreira and Lang 2006) postulates that insulin resistance may have developed during periods of food deprivation by reducing the utilisation of glucose by muscles, and favouring other organs to use the glucose instead, such as the brain. When food suddenly becomes available and a sedentary lifestyle lowers the amount of physical activity, a pathological decrease in the utilisation of glucose occurs. The generally accepted model explains that the adoption of a sedentary lifestyle and high calorific intake has resulted in an obesity epidemic, and the related type 2 diabetes prevalence rates. However, as Scheper-Hughes (2006) argues, given there is no evidence for this gene yet, this is an example of bad anthropology combined with bad genetics. It simplifies or ignores the bio-social, socio-economic, and political interactions that take place, and results in people being blamed for their illnesses. Fee has called this a 'racialising narrative…' with a '…unclear, scientific hypothesis…' (2006: 2990). Neel (1962) even revisited this 'Thrift Gene' theory because of the ways in which ambiguity, uncertainties, and multifactorial contexts are necessarily needed when discussing a compound effect of gene–environment relationships.

Despite the sheer *uncertainty* behind the genetic science in this area, the coupling of South Asian as a racial category and genetic modelling has led to a form of discursive glossing, which performs the function of creating certainty out of uncertainty. For example, Gholap et al. tell us that 'South Asians are more insulin resistant than White Europeans … although the reasons are not very clear … it is thought to be mainly related to increased adiposity, central obesity … and high body fat percentage' (2011: 47). Again, a recent review of studies by Hartley (2014) finds no additional evidence for high-risk factors that might be yielded in genetic risk profiling. I have called these liminal discursive spaces 'certain uncertainties in diabetes causality' (Keval 2015: 6) because they perform the function of knowledge production at the representational level. Whilst social contexts, culture, 'ethnic' behavioural mechanisms (as represented in discourse), all have a powerful unpredictability and uncertainty attached to them, they can be discursively contained within the parameters of static notions of culture, ethnicity, and normative positions of 'healthy lifestyles'. This process is what the book has been attempting to unpack and problematise. Genetic science, on the contrary, provides a series of supposedly incontestable 'truths' because of its representation as value-free and objective, albeit in reality, these issues are far from uni-dimensional or polarised.

While some authors would argue that these genetic understandings of human life present new spaces of agency and identity formulation (Novas and Rose 2000a), I would contend that at the intersection with race, ethnicity, and health, these spaces are somewhat overstated, especially when material and socio-economic conditions (Link and Mckinlay 2009) are taken into account. Bhopal's (2013) attempt at bringing together gene–environment factors in order to somehow solve the epidemiological puzzle of South Asian diabetes is laudable. However, it is problematic in its inclusion of vague and somewhat stereotype perpetuating tropes, such as 'cultural values' and food in South Asian groups. In-depth research has shown time and again that the consumption and management do not take place within a cultural container, sealed off from other social and economic contexts. Rather, they are fully contingent, dynamic, and culturally fluid markers of social negotiation. Thus, we are presented with both a culturally mediated form of deviance, which may result in higher rates of diabetes, plus a genetic predisposition that results in a higher vulnerability to the disease. Neither of these routes has particularly firm foundations, but they are, indeed, very much a part of the fabric of knowledge maintenance and health interventions. This liminal space of 'uncertain-certainty' reveals itself to be a site of particular ideological and practical concern, especially where people are categorised with associated 'high-risk' labels. The impacts on people's lives are far from solely symbolic, and I develop this line of argument in more detail in Chap. 9.

Conclusion

It is possible to argue that health sciences discourse has constructed what can be termed a 'South Asian diabetic risk', through a variety of ideas, including genetic predisposition to insulin resistance (McKeigue et al. 1992; Bhopal 2013; Gholap et al. 2011), primary metabolic effects (Abate and Chandalia 2003; Zimmett and Thomas 2003), and 'lifestyle' and 'cultural factors', such as sedentary lives and inappropriate nutrition (Gupta et al. 1995; BHF 2001; Naeem 2003). Through these discourses, there is a particular risk identity being shaped, which is informed by research and practice treating 'ethnicity' and 'culture' as fixed and static entities. Situating diabetes and ethnicity firmly within the social and cultural domains in which they are experienced, the overlapping mechanisms of identity forming and sustenance allows them to be interwoven into health experience. In the following chapter, I briefly outline how I accessed the people in the study and their stories.

References

Abate, N., & Chandalia, M. (2001). Ethnicity and type 2 diabetes: Focus on Asian Indians. *Journal of Diabetes Complications, 15*(6), 320–327.

Abate, N., & Chandalia, M. (2003). The impact of ethnicity on type 2 diabetes. *Journal of Diabetes and Its Complications, 17*, 39–58.

Ahmad, W. I. U. (1993). *'Race' and health in contemporary Britain*. Buckingham: Open University Press.

Ahmad, W. I. U., & Bradby, H. (2007). Locating ethnicity and health: Exploring concepts and contexts. *Sociology of Health & Illness, 29*(6), 795–810. Available at: http://www.ncbi.nlm.nih.gov/pubmed/17986016. Accessed 13 Nov 2014.

Ali, K., Kalra, V. S., & Sayyid, B. (2006). *A postcolonial people – South Asians in Britain*. London: Hurst and Co.

Atkinson, P. (1984). Training for certainty. *Social Science and Medicine, 19*, 949–956.

Bhatt, A., & Dickinson, R. (1992). An analysis of health education materials for minority communities by cultural and linguistic group. *Health Education Journal, 51*(2), 72–77.

Bhopal, R. (2013). A four-stage model explaining the higher risk of type 2 diabetes mellitus in South Asians compared with European populations. *Diabetic Medicine, 30*(1), 35–42. doi:10.1111/dme.12016.

Bhopal, R., & White, M. (1993). Health promotion for ethnic minorities: Past, present and future. In W. I. U. Ahmad (Ed.), *'Race' and health in contemporary Britain*. Buckingham: Open University Press.

Bliss, C. (2011). Racial taxonomy in genomics. *Social Science and Medicine, 73*, 1019–1027.

Bloch, A., Neal, S., & Solomos, J. (2013). *Race, multiculture and social policy*. Basingstoke: Palgrave Macmillan.

Brah, A. (2006). The Asian in Britain. In N. Ali, V. S. Kalra, & S. Sayyid (Eds.), *A postcolonial people – South Asians in Britain* (pp. 35–61). London: Hurst and Company.

British Heart Foundation. (2001). *Coronary heart disease: Statistics: Diabetes supplement*. London: BHF.

Bunton, R., & Burrows, R. (1995). Consumption and health in the 'epidemiological' clinic of late modern medicine. In R. Bunton, S. Nettleton, & R. Burrows (Eds.), *The sociology of health promotion – Critical analyses of consumption, lifestyle and risk* (pp. 206–222). London: Routledge.

Bunton, R., Nettleton, S., & Burrows, R. (1995). *The sociology of health promotion*. London: Routledge.

Cantle, T. (2012). *Interculturalism – The new era of cohesion and diversity*. London: Palgrave Macmillan.

Castel, R. (1991). From dangerousness to risk. In G. Burchell, C. Gordon, & P. Miller (Eds.), *The Foucault effect: Studies in governmentality* (pp. 281–298). Chicago: The University of Chicago Press.

Department of Health/Medical Research Council. Research Advisory Committees on Diabetes. (2002). *Current and future research on diabetes: A review for the Department of Health and the Medical Research Council*. Crown Copyright.

Diabetes UK. (2003). Cultural evolution. Diabetes Update, Winter 2003. http://www.diabetes.org.uk/update/winter03/evo.htm. Accessed 25 Jun 2004.

Farrar, M. (2004). Social movements and the struggle over 'race'. In M. J. Todd & G. Taylor (Eds.), *Democracy and participation-popular protest and new social movements*. London: Merlin Press.

Farrar, M., Robinson, S., Valli, Y., & Wetherley, P. (2012). *Islam in the West- key issues in multiculturalism*. Basingstoke: Palgrave Macmillan.

Ferreira, M., & Lang, G. (2006). *Indigenous peoples and diabetes: Community empowerment and wellness*. Durham: Carolina Academic Press.

Flynn, R., & Craig, G. (2012). Policy, politics and practice: A historical review and its relevance to current debates. In G. Craig, K. Atkin, S. Chattoo, & R. Flynn (Eds.), *Understanding 'race' and ethnicity: Theory, history, policy, practice*. Bristol: Policy Press.

Foucault, M. (1972). *Archaeology of knowledge*. London: Routledge.

Fox, R. C. (1980). The evolution of medical uncertainty. *The Millbank Memorial Quarterly. Health and Society, 58*(1), 1–49.

Fox, R. C. (2007). Medical uncertainty revisited. In G. L. Albrecht, R. Fitzpatrick, & S. C. Scrimshaw (Eds.), *The handbook of social studies in health and medicine* (pp. 409–425). London: Sage.

Gholap, N., Davies, M., Patel, K., Sattar, N., & Khunti, K. (2011). Type 2 diabetes and cardiovascular disease in South Asians. *Primary Care Diabetes, 5*, 45–56.

Gilbert, T. J., Percy, C. A., Sugarman, J. R., Benson, L., & Percy, C. (1992). Obesity among Navajo adolescents. Relationship to dietary intake and blood pressure. *American Journal of Diseases of Children, 146*(3), 289–295.

Gupta, S., de Belder, A., & O'Hughes, L. (1995). Avoiding premature coronary deaths in Asians in Britain: Spend now on prevention or pay later for treatment. *British Medical Journal, 311*, 1035–1036.

Hales, C. N., & Barker, D. J. (2001). The thrifty pheno-type hypothesis. *British Medical Bulletin, 60*, 5–20.

Ham, C. (2009). *Health policy*. Basingstoke: Palgrave Macmillan.

Ham, C., Dixon, A., & Brooke, B. (2012). *Transforming the delivery of health and social care: The case for fundamental change*. London: The Kings Fund.

Hartley, K. (2014). The genomic contribution to diabetes, briefing note: Diabetes, genomics and public health. PHG Foundation. http://www.phg-foundation.org/file/15592/. Accessed 2 Jul 2014.

Hill, J. (2006). Management of diabetes in South Asian communities in the UK. *Nursing Standard, 20*(25), 57–64.

Hu, F. (2011). Globalization of diabetes: The role of diet, lifestyle, and genes. *Diabetes Care, 34*, 1249–1257.

Hu, F. B., van Damm, R. M., & Liu, S. (2001). Diet and risk of type II diabetes: The role of types of fat and carbohydrate. *Diabetologia, 44*, 805–817.

Johnson, M. R. D. (1993). Equal opportunities in service delivery: Responses to a changing population? In W. I. U. Ahmad (Ed.), *'Race' and health in contemporary Britain*. Buckingham: Open University Press.

Keval, H. (2014). From 'multiculturalism' to 'interculturalism' – A commentary on the impact of de-racing and de-classing the debate. *New Diversities, 16*(2), 125–139. ISSN 2199-8116.

Keval, H. (2015). Risky cultures to risky genes: The racialised discursive construction of South Asian genetic diabetes risk. *New Genetics and Society*. doi: 10.1080/14636778.2015.1036155.

Khunti, K., Kumar, S., & Brodie, J. (2009). *Diabetes UK and South Asian Health Foundation recommendations on diabetes research priorities for British South Asians*. London: Diabetes UK.

Kings Fund. (2015). How much money does the NHS need? Available at: http://www.kingsfund.org.uk/projects/verdict/how-much-money-does-nhs-need Accessed 7 May 2015.

Kyriakides, A., & Virdee, S. (2003). Migrant labour, racism and the British National Health Service. *Ethnicity and Health, 8*(4), 282–305.

Lentin, A., & Titley, G. (2011). *The crises of multiculturalism – Racism in a neoliberal age*. London: Zed Books.

Link, C. L., & McKinlay, J. B. (2009). Disparities in the prevalence of diabetes: Is it race/ethnicity or socioeconomic status? Results from the Boston Area. *Ethnicity & Disease, 19*(3), 288–292.

Manson, J. E., Rimm, E. B., Stampfer, M. J., Colditz, G. A., Willett, W. C., Krolewski, A. S., Rossner, B., Hennekens, C. H., & Speizer, F. E. (1991). Physical activity and incidence of non-insulin dependent diabetes mellitus in women. *Lancet, 338*, 774–778.

Matheson, L. M., Donnigan, M. G., Hole, D., & Gillis, C. R. (1985). Incidence of colorectal, breast and lung cancer in a Scottish Asian population. *Health Bulletin (Scotland), 43*(5), 245–249.

McGregor, S. (2001). Neoliberalism and health care. *International Journal of Consumer Studies, 25*(2), 82–89.

McKeigue, P., Miller, G. J., & Marmot, M. G. (1989). Coronary heart disease in South Asians overseas – A review. *Journal of Clinical Epidemiology, 42*, 597–609.

McKeigue, P. M., Shah, B., & Marmot, M. G. (1991). Relation of central obesity and insulin resistance with high diabetes prevalence and cardiovascular risk in South Asians. *Lancet, 337*, 382–386.

McKeigue, P. M., Pierpont, T., Ferne, J. E., & Marmot, M. G. (1992). Relationship of glucose intolerance and hyperinsulinemia to body fat pattern in South Asians and Europeans. *Diabetologia, 35*, 785–791.

McNaughton, D. (2013). 'Diabesity' down under: Overweight and obesity as cultural signifiers for type 2 diabetes mellitus. *Critical Public Health, 23*(3), 274–288. doi:10.1080/09581596.2013.766671.

Mills, C. W. (1959). *The sociological imagination.* New York: Oxford University Press.

Misra, A., Chowbey, P., Makkar, N. K., et al. (2009). Consensus statement for diagnosis of obesity, abnormal obesity and the metabolic syndrome for Asian Indians and recommendations for physical activity, medical and surgical management. *Journal of the Association of Physicians of India, 57*, 163–170.

Montoya, M. J. (2011). *Making the Mexican diabetic: Race, science, and the genetics of inequality.* London: University of California Press.

Murji, K. (2008). Mis-taken identity: Being and not being Asian, African and British. *Migrations & Identities, 1*(2), 17–32.

Naeem, A. G. (2003). The role of culture and religion in the management of diabetes: A study of Kashmiri men in Leeds. *The Journal for the Royal Society for the Promotion of Health, 123*(2), 110–116.

National Institute for Health Care and Excellence. (2012a). Group and individual-level interventions to prevent type 2 diabetes among people at high risk. Available at: http://pathways.nice.org.uk/pathways/preventing-type-2-diabetes#path=view%3A/pathways/preventing-type-2-diabetes/group-and-individual-level-interventions-to-prevent-type-2-diabetes-among-people-at-high-risk.xml&content=view-node%3Anodes-encouraging-people-to-be-physically-active. Accessed 7 May 2015.

National Institute for Health Care and Excellence. (2012b). Healthy diet and exercise key to reducing the risk of type 2 diabetes. New and Features. 12 Jul 2012. Available at: https://www.nice.org.uk/news/article/healthy-diet-and-exercise-key-to-reducing-the-risk-of-type-2-diabetes. Accessed 7 May 2015.

National Institute for Health Care and Excellence. (2012c). Preventing type 2 diabetes: Risk identification and interventions for individuals at high risk.

NICE guidelines [PH38]. Available at: http://www.nice.org.uk/guidance/ph38. Accessed 7 May 2015.

Nazroo, J., & Karlsen, S. (2002). Agency and structure: The impact of ethnic identity and racism on the health of ethnic minority people. *Sociology of Health & Illness, 24*(1), 1–20.

Neel, J. V. (1962). Diabetes mellitus: A thrifty genotype rendered detrimental by 'progress'. *American Journal of Human Genetics, 14*, 353–362.

Novas, C., & Rose, R. (2000a). Genetic risk and the birth of the somatic individual. In M. Fraser & M. Greco (Eds.), *The Body-A reader* (pp. 237–241). London: Routledge.

Novas, C., & Rose, N. (2000b). Genetic risk and the birth of the somatic individual. *Economy and Society, 29*(4), 485–513.

O'Brien, M. (1995). Health and lifestyle a critical mess? Notes on the dedifferentiation of health. In R. Bunton, S. Nettleton, & R. Burrows (Eds.), *The sociology of health promotion critical analyses of consumption, lifestyle and risk* (pp. 191–205). London: Routledge.

Oldroyd, J., Banerjee, M., Heald, A., & Cruickshank, K. (2005). Diabetes and ethnic minorities. *Postgraduate Medical Journal, 81*, 486–490. doi:10.1136/pgmj.2004.029124.

Patel, N. (1993). Healthy margins, Black elders' care-models, policies and prospects. In W. I. U. Ahmad (Ed.), *'Race' and health in contemporary Britain*. Buckingham: Open University Press.

Pitcher, B. (2009). *The politics of multiculturalism – Race and racism in contemporary Britain*. Basingstoke: Palgrave Macmillan.

Ramachandran, A., Chamukuttan, S., Shetty, A. S., & Nanditha, A. (2013). Primary prevention of type 2 diabetes in South Asians -challenges and the way forward. *Diabetic Medicine, 30*, 26–34.

Ricci-Cabello, I., Ruiz-Pérez, I., Olry de Labry-Lima, A., & Márquez-Calderón, S. (2010). Do social inequalities exist in terms of the prevention, diagnosis, treatment, control and monitoring of diabetes? A systematic review. *Health and Social Care in the Community, 18*(6), 572–587. doi:10.1111/j.1365-2524.2010.00960.x.

Rocheron, Y. (1988). The Asian mother and baby campaign: The construction of ethnic minorities health needs. *Critical Social Policy, 22*, 4–23.

Rock, M. (2005). Figuring out type 2 diabetes through genetic research: Reckoning kinship and the origins of sickness. *Anthropology & Medicine, 12*(2), 115–127.

Salway, S., Platt, L., Harriss, K., & Chowbey, P. (2007). Long-term health conditions and disability living allowance: Exploring ethnic differences and similarities in access. *Sociology of Health & Illness, 29*(6), 907–930. doi:10.1111/j.1467-9566.2007.01044.x. ISSN 0141-9889.

Salway, S., Turner, D., Ghazala, M., Carter, L., Skinner, J., Bushara, B., Gerrish, K., & Ellison, G. (2013). High quality healthcare commissioning: Obstacles and opportunities for progress on race equality, Better Health Briefing 28, Race Equality Foundation. http://www.better-health.org.uk/sites/default/files/briefings/downloads/briefing%2028%20final.pdf

Scheper-Hughes, N. (2006). Diabetes and genocide-beyond the thrifty gene. In M. Ferreira & G. Lang (Eds.), *Indigenous peoples and diabetes: Community empowerment and wellness*. Durham: Carolina Academic Press.

Schonfeld, D. J., Behall, K. M., Bhathema, S. J., Reiser, S., & Revett, K. R. (1987). A study on Asian Indian men and American vegetarians: Indications of a racial predisposition to glucose intolerance. *American Journal of Clinical Nutrition, 46*, 955–961.

Schubert, L., Gallegos, D., Foley, W., & Harrison, C. (2012). Re-imagining the 'social' in the nutrition sciences. *Public Health Nutrition, 15*(2), 352–359. Available at: http://www.ncbi.nlm.nih.gov/pubmed/21729468. Accessed 13 Nov 2014.

Sevak, L., McKeigue, P. M., & Marmot, M. G. (1994). Relationship of hyper-insulinemia to dietary intake in South Asian and European men. *American Journal of Clinical Nutrition, 59*, 1069–1074.

Shafrir, E. (1996). Development and consequences of insulin resistance: Lessons from animals with hyperinsulinemia. *Diabetes and Metabolism, 22*, 122–131.

Silman, A., Loysen, E., De Graff, W., et al. (1985). High dietary fat intake and cigarette smoking as risk factors for ischaemic heart disease in Bangladeshi male immigrants in East London. *Journal of Epidemiology and Community Health, 39*, 301–303.

Stone, M., et al. (2005). Empowering patients with diabetes: A qualitative primary care study focusing on South Asians in Leicester, UK. *Family Practice, 22*, 647–652.

Stone, M. A., Patel, N., Amin, S., Daly, H., Carey, M. E., Khunti, K., et al. (2013). Developing and initially evaluating two training modules for healthcare providers, designed to enhance cultural diversity awareness and cultural competence in diabetes. *Diversity and Equality in Health and Care, 10*(3), 177–184.

Yajnik, C. S. (2001). The insulin resistance epidemic in India: Foetal origins, later lifestyle, or both? *Nutrition Reviews, 59*, 1–9.

Zimmett, P., & Thomas, C. R. (2003). Genotype, obesity and cardiovascular disease – Has technical and social advancement outstripped evolution? *Journal of Internal Medicine, 254*, 114–125.

5

Method

The data I present in this book was generated using in-depth and semi-structured interviews, and ethnographic work in several locations in England. Twenty interviews took place in four cities in England, two of which were large, multicultural urban centres with high concentrations of South Asian groups, Hindu Gujaratis specifically. In addition, I undertook visits to community centres, places of worship, and participants' homes. The aim of the book is not just to present voices of South Asian people with diabetes—such renderings have now become popular in research and policy—though this is an integral component in healthcare. Rather, I intend to set these voices against the backdrop of the discursive, racialised construction of diabetes risk among these Black and minority groups. The individuals I interviewed and groups I participated in and observed were Hindu in faith, and Gujarati in their cultural and linguistic placement. This study used purposive (Strauss and Corbin 1990) and snowball sampling (Hughes et al. 1995) to recruit participants and generate data. Nineteen type 2 diabetic and one type 1 diabetic Hindu Gujaratis were interviewed, with ages ranging from forty to eighty-eight (eight women and twelve men). I gained access to community leaders and other 'gatekeepers', who facilitated my presence at a number of gatherings in local temples and community centres.

© The Editor(s) (if applicable) and The Author(s) 2016   **87**
H. Keval, *Health, Ethnicity and Diabetes*,
DOI 10.1057/978-1-137-45703-5_5

'A Story ... Not THE Story'

Qualitative approaches facilitate the elaboration of different dimensions on which the social world operates, by emphasising the 'understandings, experiences and imaginings of our research participants ... and the significance of the meanings they generate' (Mason 2002: 1). As Riessman tells us, this is 'a story that shines light on certain objects of identity and leaves others in the shadow' (2001: 81). In acknowledging that there may be an infinite number of alternate tellings of experience, we can situate the generation of these understandings of diabetes experience in a temporal, historical, and situated context. Being a qualitative project which also situates experiences as part of the experiential resistances to discursive constructions, the book is not overly concerned with the notion of 'generalisation'. Rather than trying to establish whether or not people within a community are 'typical', it is more important to explore how, for example, people's diabetes management can be related to a broader range of experiences and discourses (Bryman 1988). The richness comes not just from what is happening in the micro details of people's lives and thinking, but also from those processes occurring in overarching systems of knowledge-making, such as epidemiology, race-health science, diabetes interventions, and social scientific analyses of race.

Diabetes: Not a Lone Project

Most of the twenty interviews took place in private homes, and more often than not, there was a third person present, usually an immediate relative. In many cases, the interview situation was characterised by this 'triad' dynamic. Contrary to Boeije's (2004) suggestion that this 'third' person decreases validity, here, it was seen as a resource for the study, which could be utilised for a rich account of the socially and culturally embedded diabetic experience. This seemed an appropriate strategy since the management of type 2 diabetes was rarely a lone biographical project, but rather, a personal and social activity carried out in the context of relationships (Peyrot et al. 1987). People were aided by significant others in complex webs of knowledge, belief, and products, so it seemed appropriate that a qualitative and situated sociology could engage in these relations rather than negate or ignore their value.

Why Hindu Gujaratis?

My research interests have centred on the experiences of South Asians in the UK in general, with a special focus on health and illness. These interests also extend to the role of traditional and lay beliefs, and the ways in which migration experiences, and the general cultural experience, or expressions of 'cultural navigation' (Ballard 1994) manifest themselves in everyday life. For this reason, individuals describing themselves as belonging to a particular faith group—Hindus—were chosen. The age criteria were chosen for two reasons. It has been documented that there are generational differences in experiences between migrants of different age groups, with a variety of factors playing roles in how individuals traverse the varying cultural universes, employing linguistic, cultural, religious, and social techniques to accomplish this (Bhachu 1986). Because of this distinction, I focused on the experiences of first-generation migrants from South Asia and East Africa, in order not to homogenise groups which have distinct characteristic experiences. The second reason for choosing this age group is linked to the nature of type 2 diabetes. As it is also known as 'mature' or 'later onset' diabetes, the age at which diagnosis takes place is usually around 40 years, although data now indicates it is appearing in people much younger than this (Ehtisham et al. 2000). As already shown by numerous authors (Visram 2002; Ballard 1994; Hill 1969; Hiro 1992), there is a long history of migration from South Asian countries to the UK. Many of the participants talked to me about their lives in this country and of life in a new land, where hostility and aggression were often the norm. However, they also talked about some aspects of their lives both in India and in Africa, including the process of settling in the UK. These experiences are inextricably connected to the overall experience the book explores—diabetes being one aspect of this range.

Gujarat

Gujarat, a state in India, lies north of Mumbai on its West coast. Its location on the coast made it an ideal place for trade routes to a variety of locations to be set up, including to Africa and the Middle East. Internal trading routes also benefited from Gujarat, as archaeological evidence demonstrates evidence of trading with Mesopotamia in the second millennium BCE, and many later references during Buddhist, Muslim, and Hindu presences to the thriving culture of trade, commerce, hard work, frugal living, and entrepreneurial entities (Dwyer 1994). These traditions continued as the nineteenth century progressed, with Gujarati migration being reinforced first by the sheer force of overseas trade, and second, by the British colonial expansion into East Africa, bringing with it many socio-economic and political as well as cultural changes (Warrier 1994). Many of the participants locate their experiences within this historically and identity-centred landscape—a concept Ballard (1994) discusses in detail—the *desh pardesh* phenomenon (literally, 'home from home', or 'at home abroad').

As a South Asian diasporic entity, Hindu Gujaratis form part of a hugely diverse general South Asian global movement, which takes in several temporal as well as global-spatial arenas (Jacobsen and Kumar 2004). The variation in religious and cultural frameworks is extensive, as is the wide-ranging settlement patterns over time and space. In the 2011 census (ONS 2012), 817,000 people self-identified as Hindu (1.5 % of the England and Wales population), but unfortunately, there are no official population figures for people who then also identify as having some form of identity affiliation with Gujarat. Dwyer (2004) reports estimates of approximately 500,000, again stressing the lack of census data, while Bevan (2013) makes a general statement about the city of Leicester having the largest population of Gujaratis outside of the state of Gujarat, India. Given the global movement of these diasporic groups over the last 150 years (Jacobsen and Kumar 2004) and the substantial constitution of this in terms of Gujarati people, the dearth of systematic census information is interesting, especially given the relationship between the two main phases of emigration from South Asia (Vertovec 2000) is intimately colonial and postcolonially configured—either through independence of the 'home' country from imperial rule or from 1947 (Indian independence) onwards, owing to the search for opportunities in work and education.

The Hindu Gujarati section of the British South Asian population is comparatively under-researched. Most research which has purported to examine issues related to health and ethnicity in the South Asian population bases its distinction between groups solely on national and intra-national boundaries—hence Indian, Pakistani, and Bangladeshi groups. However, this is oversimplifying a complex issue. The homogenising of groups which are clearly distinctive in terms of culture, language, social and community networks, and migration histories does little justice to the experiences people have. There is very little distinction given to varying organising principles, such as caste, which, as a global diasporic organisational and logistic phenomenon, has very different manifestations according to the caste characteristics. Nor is there much distinction in the literature reviewed (Ballard 1994 is an exception) between British South Asians from India, and those who arrived in the UK from Africa—both groups who have had different socio-cultural experiences. As discussed earlier, the UK has a long history of migrant relationships with South Asians from India, Pakistan, and parts of Africa (Murji 2008).

The literature on the experience of diabetes seldom ventures into in-depth studies of minority groups, though the last decade has seen interesting development (e.g. Greenhalgh et al. 1998, 2005; Ferreira and Lang 2006). This is in stark contrast to the traditional epidemiological studies, based on data from a variety of population studies. While there is an abundance of studies which look at the experiences of White people in the UK, again, in-depth research into the British South Asian communities is lacking (exceptions are Kelleher and Islam 1996; Greenhalgh et al. 1998; Lawton et al. 2005, 2006a, b; Stone et al. 2013; Chattoo and Ahmad 2004). Indeed, Greenhalgh's work on 'sharing stories' included Gujarati speakers and the use of bilingual health advocates leading Gujarati groups in health education. The notion of 'sharing stories'—a way of engaging with non-English-speaking diabetics—through user groups and bilingual advocates can lead to 'learning, empowerment and change' (2005: 632). As Ferreira and Lang (2006) have demonstrated, it is possible to gain access to people's cultural worlds, in the context of their history and culture in symbolic and practical terms, and locate health ideas, solutions, and avenues for better lives within the social and cultural lives they lead.

Hagey (1984) discusses incorporating cultural knowledge into health education in Toronto among the Aanishinaabe people, while Greenhalgh et al.'s (1998) earlier work emphasised how beliefs in their Bangladeshi sample could be used effectively in culturally sensitive diabetes education. These models frame diabetes in terms of a series of historical and political forces, which have brought about the decimation of traditional cultures through power relations and inequalities, resulting in unequal access to a range of resources (Ferreira and Lang 2006). These processes include limitation of access to appropriate and culturally traditional food and diet resources (Lang 2006) and internalisation of the construction of a 'genetic' risk (Scheper-Hughes 2006). These provide insights into the political and historical forces that impinge on what people do within the diabetes experience, how they manage their illness, and the kinds of socio-cultural contexts people operate within. These studies progress the area further by creating—with indigenous groups—programmes of health awareness, which take as their focus their own history, life experiences, systems of traditional knowledge, including herbs, and foods (Korn and Ryser 2006).

As Ferreira and Lang (2006) vehemently argue in their 'local knowledges' and community empowerment thesis, accounting for the histories of people where oppression and subjugation have been central to people's lives over generations is key to understanding not just 'how' questions in diabetes, but also 'why' questions concerning diabetes in indigenous populations. Although the people in this study may not be categorised as 'indigenous' (this is a contestable concept in any case) and not perhaps strictly categorised as 'oppressed' (though this is infinitely debatable), there are some interesting possibilities in looking to narratives and life worlds within the diabetes experience which help to facilitate an understanding of wider historical and discursive forces.

'Researcher' and 'Researched' Roles: The Politics of Minding and Bridging the Gap

The process of talking with, interviewing, observing, and learning about the issues that were important to people involved the interconnection of roles, between what have been traditionally viewed as the researcher–

researched identities. Gunaratnam (2003) highlighted the problems of interviewing across difference by posing the question of how White researchers can somehow bridge the gap between themselves and the minorities they want to study, by running the risk of what Anderson (1993) called distorting sociological accounts in terms of race, gender, and class. It would be overly simplistic to regard this study as unproblematic in this aspect, simply because the interviewer shares certain dimensions of his identity with the study group. There are issues here related to constructions of 'authenticity' and their impact on the research. Since no two research interviews will be identical, there are bound to be many issues at play while the production of the interview is underway. These are important considerations, and as Smaje (1995) has warned against 'ideological categories', so Gunaratnam (2003) warns against 'categorical thinking'. Rather than emulating some model of natural science by attempting to control variables which, in a socially constructed reality, are beyond control, this study hopes to actively engage in the dynamic processes involved in the ways in which two identities come together, sometimes connecting, and at other times, clashing. It is perhaps in the process of negotiating the interaction of differences and similarities that the lived experience of a person with diabetes can be understood. As Song and Parker state, the 'unfolding of the researcher's and interviewee's cultural identities is central to the ways in which the researcher and researched position themselves in relation to the "other" ' (1995: 243).

As someone who locates parts of his own identity as intersecting with multiple aspects of the participant's identities, I found it to be interesting and important to acknowledge these lines of connection. I have explored these connections—'cultural validations' in detail elsewhere (Keval 2009), and regard them to be an important and integral component of empirical research—especially in work which explores ideas of difference. There are no clear lines demarcating what 'types' of identity matching or un-matching will lead to robust and rich research. Rather, the idea of 'cultural validations' helps us to at least acknowledge the intersecting, mixing, and contingent manner of researcher–researched identity-making. If we accept that all identities are continuous processes (Hall 1992), then there can be no 'fixed' state of connecting with participants, and research must work with the view that, at any given time, there will be multiple connections and disconnections between the involved. The use of language is part of this process. The decision to conduct the study in both Gujarati and English was based on entering the 'cultural domain' (Silverman 1993) of the people who were willingly opening their homes and lives to me. This 'life world' (Schutz 1966) was constituted, in part, by the language that was spoken and was crucial to understanding and answering the research questions.

The process of social action requires language to facilitate it, and accepting the role of language as a system of symbols and gestures to communicate universes of meaning requires acceptance of its crucial and central role. Hence, the importance given to the process of 'cultural validation', for it is mainly—though not entirely—through linguistic connection that this process of screening, acceptance, or rejection takes place. During the fieldwork, were I not able to speak the language as well as converse about commonalities in histories, then access may not have been gained so easily; the kinds of topics discussed may have been different; the level of disclosure may have varied; and the vital social connection which is such a powerful theme here may have been lost. This, of course, does not necessarily mean that similar research by someone who was not fluent in this South Asian language would produce fewer insights; simply that the research outcome would be different, as would the relationship between the researcher and the researched. The importance of language, of course, has been long established by anthropologists, but sociologists undertaking this kind of work have also relied on having the linguistic connection (e.g. Kelleher and Islam 1996; Reed 2003; Bradby 2002). In many ways, being able to conduct the interviews in a language most familiar to the participant, but having the option to also conduct them in English performed a useful conceptual function. On a practical and methodological level, it made the participant more comfortable; but on another level, it symbolised the relationship which first-generation migrants have with a 'host' country. The process of translation has been described in some detail by specialists elsewhere (Birbili 2000), and in many ways, is peripheral to this study, because the translation is not simply of words and how they constitute language, but rather, of how these words constitute social action. Bradby (2002) has succinctly emphasised the importance of language and linguistic competencies, or at least, the cooperation with linguistic expertise when working in the arena of ethnicity and health. I would extend this argument further, and argue that both this competency and a critical appraisal of identities are required for the research to be able to translate meanings—as created and sustained by participants. This means that not only might language be important, but the cultural and social complexities of context need to be understood, in ways which will allow a connection to participants to be set up and for the contingent nature of field relations to be facilitated (Ryen 2008).

Part 2 of the book presents the different ways in which participants talked about living with diabetes and negotiating the social fabric into which their identities were woven. By presenting these aspects of people's experiences, the discursive constructions of risk which I have attempted to signpost in the preceding chapters can be set against the fluid and dynamic cultural, ethno-religious, and biographical resources that people called upon in their negotiations.

References

Anderson, M. L. (1993). Studying across difference: Race, class, and gender in qualitative research. In J. H. Stanfield & M. Dennis (Eds.), *Race and ethnicity in research methods*. Newbury Park: Sage.

Ballard, R. (1994). *Desh Pardesh: The South Asian presence in Britain*. London: Hurst.

Bevan, J. D. (2013). *There are close links between Britain and Gujarat*. Speech by the British High Commissioner to India Sir James Bevan KCMG at the inaugural session of the Vibrant Gujarat Global Investors Summit. Foreign and Commonwealth Office. 11th Jan 2013. Available at: https://www.gov.uk/government/speeches/there-are-close-links-between-britain-and-gujarat

Bhachu, P. (1986). *Twice migrants*. London: Tavistock.

Birbili, M. (2000). Translating from one language to another, Social Research Update, Issue 31.

Boeije, H. R. (2004). And then there were three: Self-presentational styles and the presence of the partner as a third person in the interview. *Field Methods, 16*(1), 3–22.

Bradby, H. (2002). Translating culture and language: A research note on multilingual settings. *Sociology of Health & Illness, 24*(6), 842–855.

Bryman, A. (1988). *Quantity and quality in social research*. London: Unwin Hyman.

Chattoo, S., & Ahmad, W. I. U. (2004). The meaning of cancer: Illness, biography and social identity. In D. Kelleher & G. Leavey (Eds.), *Identity and health* (pp. 19–36). London: Routledge.

Dwyer, R. (1994). Caste, religion and sect in Gujarat: Followers of Vallabhacharya and Swaminarayan. In R. Ballard (Ed.), *Desh Pardesh: The South Asian presence in Britain*. London: Hurst.

Dwyer, R. (2004). The Swaminarayan movement. In K. A. Jacobsen & P. Kumar (Eds.), *South Asians in the diaspora – Histories and religious traditions* (pp. 180–199). Leiden: Brill.

Ehtisham, S., Barrett, T. G., & Shaw, N. J. (2000). Type 2 diabetes mellitus in UK children – An emerging problem. *Diabetic Medicine, 17*(12), 867–871.

Ferreira, M., & Lang, G. (2006). *Indigenous peoples and diabetes: Community empowerment and wellness*. Durham: Carolina Academic Press.

Greenhalgh, T., Helman, C., & Chowdhury, A. M. (1998). Health beliefs and folk models of diabetes in British Bangladeshis: A qualitative study. *British Medical Journal, 316*, 978–983.

Greenhalgh, T., Collard, A., & Begum, N. (2005). Sharing stories: Complex intervention for diabetes education in minority ethnic groups who do not speak English. *British Medical Journal, 330*, 628.

Gunaratnam, Y. (2003). *Researching 'race' and ethnicity: Methods, knowledge and power*. London: Sage.

Hagey, R. (1984). The phenomenon, the explanations and the responses: Metaphors surrounding diabetes in urban Canadian Indians. *Social Science and Medicine, 18*(3), 265–272.

Hall, S. (1992). New ethnicities. In J. Donald & A. Rattanasi (Eds.), *Race, culture and difference*. London: Sage.

Hill, C. (1969). *Immigration and integration*. Devon: Perganon Press.

Hiro, D. (1992). *Black British, white British*. London: Grafton Books.

Hughes, A. O., Fenton, S., & Hine, C. E. (1995). Strategies for sampling Black and ethnic minority populations. *Journal of Public Health, 17*(2), 187–192.

Jacobsen, K. A., & Kumar, P. P. (2004). *South Asians in the diaspora – Histories and religious traditions*. Leiden: Brill.

Kelleher, D., & Islam, S. (1996). 'How should live?' Bangladeshi people and noninsulin dependent diabetes. In D. Kelleher & S. Hillier (Eds.), *Researching cultural differences in health*. London: Routledge.

Keval, H. (2009). Negotiating constructions of 'insider'/'outsider' status and exploring the significance of dis/connections. *ENQUIRE (Electronic Nottingham Quarterly for Ideas, Research and Evaluation), 4, Enquire 2*(2), 215–232.

Korn, L. E., & Ryser, R. C. (2006). Burying the umbilicus. Nutrition trauma, diabetes and traditional medicine in rural West Mexico. In M. Ferreira & G. Lang (Eds.), *Indigenous peoples and diabetes: Community empowerment and wellness*. Durham: Carolina Academic Press.

Lang, G. C. (2006). 'In their tellings'. Ethnographic contexts and illness narratives. In M. Ferreira & G. Lang (Eds.), *Indigenous peoples and diabetes: Community empowerment and wellness*. Durham: Carolina Academic Press.

Lawton, J., Peel, E., Parry, O., Araoza, G., & Douglas, M. (2005). Lay perceptions of type 2 diabetes in Scotland: Bringing health services back in. *Social Science & Medicine, 60*, 1423–1435.

Lawton, J., Ahmad, N., Hanna, M., Douglas, M., & Hallowell, N. (2006a). 'I can't do any serious exercise': Barriers to physical activity amongst people of Pakistani and Indian origin with type 2 diabetes. *Health Education Research, 21*(1), 43–54.

Lawton, J., Ahmad, N., Hanna, M., Douglas, M., & Hallowell, N. (2006b). Diabetes service provision: A qualitative study of the experience and views of Pakistani and Indian patients with type 2 diabetes. *Diabetic Medicine, 23*, 1003–1007.

Mason, J. (2002). *Qualitative interviewing*. London: Sage.

Murji, K. (2008). Mis-taken identity: Being and not being Asian, African and British. *Migrations & Identities, 1*(2), 17–32.

Office for National Statistics. (2012). Religion in England and Wales 2011. Available at: http://www.ons.gov.uk/ons/dcp171776_290510.pdf

Peyrot, M., McMurry, J., & Hedges, R. (1987). Living with diabetes: The role of personal and professional knowledge in symptoms and regimen management. In J. Roth & P. Conrad (Eds.), *Research in the sociology of health care* (Vol. 6). Greenwich: Jai Press.

Reed, K. (2003). *Worlds of health: Exploring the health choices of British Asian mothers*. London: Praeger.

Riessman, C. K. (2001). Personal troubles as social issues: Narrative of infertility in context. In I. Shaw & N. Gould (Eds.), *Qualitative researching in social work*. London: Sage.

Ryen, A. (2008). Wading the field with my key informant: Exploring field relations. *Qualitative Sociology Review, 4*(3), 84–104.

Scheper-Hughes, N. (2006). Diabetes and genocide-beyond the thrifty gene. In M. Ferreira & G. Lang (Eds.), *Indigenous peoples and diabetes: Community empowerment and wellness*. Durham: Carolina Academic Press.

Schutz, A. (1966). Some structures of the life-world. In T. Luckmann (Ed.), *Phenomenology and Sociology*. London: Penguin.

Silverman, D. (1993). *Interpreting qualitative data.* London: Sage.

Smaje, C. (1995). *Health, 'race' and ethnicity: Making sense of the evidence.* London: The King's Fund.

Song, M., & Parker, D. (1995). Commonality, difference and the dynamics of disclosure in in-depth interviewing. *Sociology, 29,* 241–256.

Stone, M. A., Patel, N., Amin, S., Daly, H., Carey, M. E., Khunti, K., Davies, M. J., & Dogra, N. (2013). Developing and initially evaluating two training modules for healthcare providers, designed to enhance cultural diversity awareness and cultural competence in diabetes. *Diversity and Equality in Health and Care, 10,* 177–184.

Strauss, A., & Corbin, J. (1990). *Basics of qualitative research: Grounded theory procedures and techniques.* London: Sage.

Vertovec, S. (2000). *The Hindu diaspora: Comparative patterns.* London: Routledge.

Visram, R. (2002). *Asians in Britain: 400 years of history.* London: Pluto.

Warrier, S. (1994). Gujarati Prajapatis in London: Family roles and sociability networks. In R. Ballard (Ed.), *Desh Pardesh: The South Asian presence in Britain.* London: Hurst.

Part II

Resisting Constructions of Risk: The Counter-Narratives

The preceding chapters have laid the foundations for a critical, conceptual, and theoretical discussion of how a condition such as diabetes comes to be produced in the process of social, epidemiological, and biomedical interventions, as a category of especially high risk for South Asian people around the world. This high risk category, as we have seen, is not limited to South Asians, either in the subcontinent or in the UK. There are several 'racial' groups, defined, determined, and classified in the ethno-diabetes discourses, as being of particular risk, including the Pima Indians of Arizona, USA, (Smith-Morris 2006) and the Mexican population in the USA and Mexico (Montoya 2011). The main question which Part one presents is that, paralleling Montoya's questioning (2011), given that we are embroiled within a complex, political, social, and cultural meaning-making process of health, can the people who work within this industry ignore the discursive, racialised constructions of South Asian diabetes risk?

The variety of processes which have gone into making what is now cumulatively accomplished as 'the' diabetes burden are held to history, migration, the politics of tolerance, and the many ways in which the symbolic and practical markers demarcate that which symbolises normative order and that which appears disordered and potentially dangerous (Douglas 1966). The constructions of risk, as we have seen in Part one, move from enduring legacies of post-migration interactions with minority groups, to the health science discourse on epidemiological patterns of incidence and prevalence, and descriptions of difference taken as explanations mobilised by 'cultural' deficits (lifestyle, diet, and exercise). These formulations of South Asian diabetic risk are, on the one hand, firmly validated within a scientific legitimation assemblage, but on the other, if we shift our focus, also fundamentally impactful on the way in which we view racialised constructions. They have an impact on health policy, as well as on the groups in question, as people come to understand their condition and their own medicalised, geneticised position within frames of differential culpability. The knowledge base which results in the global discourse, and specifically with reference to analysis of South Asians in the UK, necessarily needs to be viewed as a series of 'situated knowledges' (Haraway 1988). Such knowledge is politically produced, and mediated by power relations—at times, visible, but mostly operating under the visible spectrum of *acritical* gazes. In outlining his aims and intentions for his incisive ethnography of 'Mexican diabetes', Montoya states 'I hope to stimulate discomfort in the way diabetes is currently conceived...' (2011: xxi). In a similar fashion, I am situating the previous chapters in Part one as a situational backdrop against which the participant's talk and experiences in Part two can be set, mobilised, and viewed as forms of daily, interactional, and embodied resistances. I use the term *resistance* to articulate the ways in which what people do and say about their life-embedded health condition often contrast sharply with preconceived *and* contemporary representations of minority health (Keval 2009), and as such, offer the exploration of counter-narratives.

In the process of this study, I talked with people and elicited narratives about their lives and their sense and meaning-making of diabetes. As situated, strategic accounts of their lives (Smith-Morris 2006), the people in this study narrated a variety of different facets of their lives, and managed the research encounter, mine and their identities, and the communication of selected aspects of their diabetes stories (Kleinman 1988). This section of the book begins with how people react to and think about the diagnosis of diabetes, the prescriptive requirements of exercise, and the related notions of 'appropriate' diet. In Part one, I explored some of the academic and government policy discourse around these ideas. Here, we look to what the participants say about these ideas, and what this, in turn, may indicate about these contrasting positions. In continuance of this active and dynamic use of cultural and ethnic identity, the following chapter explores the use of a variety of different help-seeking systems employed by the participants in the sample. As research has established, people do not usually either understand their bodies and health conditions in simplistic, one-dimensional ways, nor do they usually rely on one type of help. In this chapter, I look at the ways in which, as Reed (2003) in her work with British Asian mothers also shows, syncretic use of different systems in parallel with each other tells us not only something important about the specific condition and remedies, but the complex forging of new identities, sometimes called 'hybridisations'.

In a similar fashion, the use of complementary, alternative, traditional, and allopathic models of healthcare and help (Chap. 7) are not mutually exclusive nor should they be 'culturalised'. This last point echoes the remarks made in earlier chapters, that there exists, at every turn, the potential risk of turning a pattern, behaviour, utterance, or attitude into a culturally specific expression. I am not arguing that using specifics from a cultural framework is incorrect or inappropriate, but applying the notion of 'culture' as a way of grouping people for convenient analytics is, at its best, conceptually not informative, and at its worst, potentially recirculates older 'bio-race' tropes.

The penultimate chapter in this section, Chap. 8, takes the preceding notions of embedded resistance to constructions of South Asian risk, and engages them further in the dimension of biography and community. In many ways, this chapter aims to explore the connections between those ideas presented in the early chapter, related to race relations and immigration in the UK and diabetes as a condition which many South Asian people in the UK have become very familiar with and embedded with the idea and practice of 'community'. As I explain in the chapter, I use the term 'community' in as flexible and fluid way as possible, but one which also allows some purchase to be expressed in terms of how people utilise the networks of affiliation around them. Again, whilst using terms related to 'culture', I aim to avoid culturalisation. The networks, affiliation, connections, postcolonial identity links, and ethno-religious connections which people talk about and use, as well as the ones they do not talk about, are echoed in the same forms of connection which communities all over the world will use. What is specific to these groups is, first, the range of direct and indirect racialised experiences that South Asian people in the UK may have experienced, and second, the range of discursive racialised constructions of risk they have been subjected to. So, whilst the human social and cultural machinery of 'doing' aspects of health may be universal, the specific postcolonial and racialised specifics above make for a different experience of health and illness for many groups of people.

References

Douglas, M. (1966). *Purity and danger*. Harmondsworth: Penguin.
Haraway, D. (1988). Situated knowledges: The science question in feminism as a site of discourse on the privilege of partial perspective. *Feminist Studies, 14*(3), 575–599.

Keval, H. (2009). Cultural negotiations in health and illness: The experience of type 2 diabetes among Gujarati-speaking South Asians in England. *Diversity in Health and Care, 16*(4), 255–265.

Kleinman, A. (1988). *The illness narratives: Suffering, healing and the human condition.* New York: Basic Books.

Montoya, M. J. (2011). *Making the Mexican diabetic: Race, science, and the genetics of inequality.* London: University of California Press.

Reed, K. (2003). *Worlds of health: Exploring the health choices of British Asian mothers.* London: Praeger.

Smith-Morris, C. (2006). *Diabetes among the Pima: Stories of survival.* Tucson: University of Arizona Press.

6

Doing Everyday Diabetes

So far, in this book, I have maintained that there is little question about the seriousness of the impact of diabetes on people's lives worldwide, nor is there any doubt about the technical legitimacy of the bio-physiological sciences in their rendering of the issue. We can, however, discern that there is a relationship between health and illness states and the forces of knowledge production as they become mediated by networks of expert power. The way in which diabetes has been studied, and how that knowledge has been applied by a variety of expert areas, including epidemiology, generates a particular perspective of diabetes that can be queried by critical work. While North American anthropology has been quick to apply a critical gaze to the production of situated knowledge, and to render louder those voices of subjugated populations hitherto silenced (see Ferreira and Lang 2006; Fee 2006; Rock 2005), sociologists dealing in diabetes and minority groups have been less willing to take on a more critical gaze until recently (laudable health service and user intervention studies notwithstanding). With this in mind, I have tried to lay the foundations for identifying some possible ways in which people categorised and deemed to be of South Asian origin in the UK are subject to constructions of particular, racialised constructions of diabetes risk. They

© The Editor(s) (if applicable) and The Author(s) 2016
H. Keval, *Health, Ethnicity and Diabetes*,
DOI 10.1057/978-1-137-45703-5_6

are represented in the discursive constructions embedded into our daily 'health' aware lives, as 'risky bodies'.

The people I spent time with and talked with as part of the fieldwork for this study demonstrated something that ran counter to these passive, culturally deviant, ethnically monolithic, and fatalistic constructions. In their talking to me about how they 'do diabetes', a number of salient issues emerged—for example, how they came to know about their condition, nutrition and physical activity, and the everyday monitoring of blood glucose levels. This connects to much of the experiential knowledge base in existence for diabetes, but in other ways, it also shows us that the types of resources people use in multiple and interconnected ways mean that reifying blocks of people within racially and ethnically homogenous categories and applying sweeping generalisations about 'lifestyle', diet, and lack of physical activity are conceptually off the mark, and also theoretically insufficient for diabetes help provision.

Far from a passive acceptance of established and conventional allopathic diagnostic procedures, participants would use various resources to triangulate symptoms, using overseas information networks, and present these to the GP. In accordance with what social analysis has been indicating for many decades, health and 'illness behaviour' (Mechanic 1978; Helman 1990) is a complex series of ongoing and adaptable entities, situated within the lived social arena of the respondents' experience. Similarly, with nutritional ideas, people within this study would step from talking in general about what they could and should do, to being explicit about specific circumstances where blood glucose levels may be affected, and how they counter this. Health service literature abounds with research which has proceeded from conceptually limited culture-blaming theses (Gupta et al. 1995; Hill 2006; Qureshi 1989) to more complex and contextual accounts (Ahmad and Bradby 2007; Lawton et al. 2005). However, there remains a need for more substantial theoretical purchase—that is, how are these notions of activity which are so closely connected to diabetes and health management conceptualised, symbolised, and acted upon? Some of the participants felt compelled to 'admit' that members of the 'South Asian community' as a whole were not physically active enough, but insisted that they themselves were not part of this deficit. Rather than write this as a 'version' or 'construction', here, it can be framed as a performance of 'private' and 'public' accounts (Cornwell 1984). On the one hand, people reported that there was some validity to views of people not taking enough exercise to help with the illness; but on the other, there were many other things which people were doing, which constituted exercise. In addition, people in this sample of South Asians had integrated activity into their everyday lives, being very aware of the prevailing climate of exercise and nutrition promotion apparent in social and cultural media. Similarly, the monitoring of blood glucose was something which most of the respondents were acutely aware of and acted upon, having different indicators of high and low levels. Even those who had had great difficulty in comprehending the technical details and mechanics of the process were able to source local expertise to ensure monitoring. The medication regimes were not always simply taken for granted as 'tablets for life'—as some accepted—but in some cases, there was active adjustment taking place. Where a weekend of eating and socialising may have caused a peak in blood glucose, especially just before a doctors' appointment, the participants, rather than take the increased medication dose prescribed because of elevated levels, would simply continue on the old dosage to achieve stability. This demonstrates a need to maintain stability in the allopathic help-seeking environment, but also a need to resist complete surrender to the regime, and retain control of one's own body. Certainly, these embodied resistances form central components of the overall scheme of analysis in this book. Diabetes is not only a psycho-social and biomedical interface-led issue but also a fundamentally embodied one, and it is precisely through these embodied practices of help-seeking, self-regulation, monitoring, and accounting *as they intersect with official medical discourses* that counter-narratives to risk constructions are formed and acted out.

'Community'

Within this study, I refer to the notion of a 'South Asian community' to describe and characterise the people involved. However, this runs the theoretical and empirical risk of reifying what is essentially a fluid notion of collectivity and belonging. The word 'community' is used here to frame a sense of fluid sociality, where people move between groups, differentiated by utility, and social and cultural need. In this way, there is really very little that appears like a homogenous South Asian community, but rather there seem to be groups of people who given their biographical, historical, and immediately located experiences can identify with resources that help to lubricate social and personal interaction. As Cornwell (1984) underlined, simply describing at-face-value accounts of cohesion and interaction within peoples' lives is underestimating the divisions and disputes that may exist, and as raised by Bulmer (1987), leads to the idealisation of groups pictured as tight-knit and solid. 'The South Asian community' here is reflected in a shared identification with what, in this study, was connected to being Hindu Gujarati, as this seems to be one identifying factor (although not the only one). The word 'community' here is used to indicate belonging via language, country of origin, religion, and sometimes, caste. However, as is demonstrated later, these are not rigid or fixed; they have a fluidity which, far from being out of reach or control of social actions, is used dynamically and in the service of managing diabetes. The people I spoke to were migrants from both India and East Africa—two very distinct, but connected diasporic groups, each with its own linguistic, historical, ethnic, and social patterns. As Brah (2006) tells us, 'Discussions about culture must be understood within the context of the power relations amongst different groups' (2006: 35), and as such, the individuals I spoke to were characterised by this heterogeneity. Therefore, the idea of community I use in this book parallels, in many ways, Parekh's rejection of 'credit card'-based notions of identity. These formulations of having multiple identities imply that identity is a possession, fixed and objective, and is used in isolation, in given contexts. Instead, Parekh argues identities '…are forms of relationship…constantly in the making' (2007: 132). Being South Asian, a migrant, diabetic, Hindu, and also, being part of sets of wider social, local, and transnational networks were all interconnected and overlapping ways of being that were fluid and subject to change.

Finding Out About the Diagnosis

There are a variety of factors involved in a diabetic following a prescribed treatment path, or deviating from it. Kelleher (1988) consistently shows that changes in lifestyle routine affect social relationships, working life, and family patterns. These can also be influenced by factors related to socio-economic status, whereby some sections of the population may have more access to financial resources and time flexibility in order to follow their daily treatment more rigorously. Diabetics may not fully understand the complex details of their illness, and the often complicated system of monitoring and evaluating the body's state. As studies show, there are many factors involved in the active and inactive evaluation that contributes to a decision, which involves a variety of prioritising measures. Kelleher discusses the many roles and responsibilities a person may have to operate within. It may be within the parameters of these roles and the duties they hold that a diabetic will set priorities according to their needs, and which results in a particular form of treatment adherence. While medical professionals may use the terms 'compliance' and 'non-compliance', it may actually be the diabetic patient exercising individual choice, based on personal life circumstances and the bringing to the medical encounter of their own agenda in addition to the medical agenda (Kelleher 1988).

One of the initial lines of enquiry in the interviews was a question about how people found out they were diabetic. Given that over the last several years, the government and various organisations, as well as academic and health research, consistently feature people in the UK population who may have type 2 diabetes, but are not aware of it (IDF 2013; Diabetes UK 2013), it was prudent to ask about this. Research has, in the past, indicated that certain sections of the population have differential likelihoods to access help, information, and diagnostic care (Nazroo 1997). However, beyond any issues related to ethnicity or culture, investigating how people found out they had a chronic illness such as diabetes not only is inherently sociologically interesting, but also contributes to the overall intellectual puzzle before us—how do people conceptualise diabetes? What do people do in their everyday lives to manage and deal with the illness, and in what ways are these mechanisms embedded in a social context? Enquiring about how people found out about their diagnosis may then provide the beginnings not only of a story about diabetes management, but also of a road map, charting the culturally and agentively negotiated territory of health and illness management. Though finding out about the illness was usually a chance occurrence, the diagnosis was still contextualised by living with the symptoms for some time, so the process of acquiring the diagnosis and the actions and thoughts of people afterwards may illuminate the various mechanisms by which the illness was dealt with. I asked a question about how they came to know they had diabetes, and the answers were quite uniform. On the whole, participants reported how they had the usually cited symptoms of tiredness, thirst, and frequent need to urinate. Even though Dhansuk (aged 54), who has been actively involved in the community, talks with ease about diabetes, as he has experience, both in his family and through his local 'Expert patient' programme, his diagnosis was still a surprise:

> ...I used to go to the loo quite often, and I used to feel thirsty... I had an occasion to take my brother to the hospital, and I just mentioned to the nurse that I was having this sort of symptom, so she said, 'Alright let me just check your urine'. And she said, 'Did you know that you have got diabetes?' So that's how I came to know about it.

Naresh (aged 72), whose wife was also present at the interview, again found out about his condition through a routine procedure for another ailment:

> I found out about 5–6 years ago. I didn't know about the symptoms myself, but I went to have keyhole surgery on my shoulder, and had some tests, and that's when I found out about sugar levels. Otherwise, I didn't have any other symptoms.

Once symptoms have become salient and have impacted both the diabetes sufferer and others, decisions are rarely taken in isolation and a plethora of important factors are accounted for—including the stressful and anxiety-provoking effects on family members. Other participants' also had similar experiences, as well as some emotional and psychological effects, such as short tempers:

> I shout at people a lot. I lose my temper! Because of this diabetes, my temper is really short! If my wife says something to me, or my son or daughter say something, then I'm ok. I realise that I shouted for nothing. I get angry at the slightest *things*. (Pramod, 59)
> Diabetics get hot-tempered. Wives, children, all need to understand this. But they argue with him, and his blood pressure goes up. (Kishore, 59)

The onset of diabetes, then, as has been documented, had an impact on the biological, social, and the psychological realms of experience. Pramod, who is 59 and retired, living with his wife and daughter, is trying to explain his shortness of temper, which—although may be for a number of reasons—in this context indicates the meaning he attaches to this event and the significance it has for him. Kishore echoes these sentiments, and looks to the problematic interactions that can take place, calling on lay ideas of the causes of rising blood pressure. The impacts of diabetes, however, are often mitigated by factors such as being familiar with or having had some exposure to the condition, and is discussed next.

Checking the Diagnosis

Most of the diagnoses were as a result of chance—for example, during a medical check-up for another problem, blood results would reveal diabetes. This, however, was not always straightforward, as some of the respondents used a 'double check' strategy—Naresh explains how this took place:

> The level was very high when I was first tested before the surgery, and I told the GP. He didn't send me to a diabetic clinic or anything, but I wanted to know why this diabetes has happened. It was actually in India, in an article which talked about the tablets I had been taking, when I realised that the

diabetes was a side effect. Then, I went to my GP and asked him if taking this blood pressure medication might cause diabetes, and he said, 'maybe'; I said, 'no not maybe, it's true.' And I showed him the article. Then, he stopped my medication and put me on other tablets.

While one would not expect this to be a straightforward process normally, as help-seeking trajectories are invariably varied, it is interesting here how Naresh used a contact in India to send him an article, which he then presented to his GP, suggesting that the side effects of the particular tablets he had been taking may have led to diabetes. Only then was his medication changed. This demonstrates that though usage of healthcare and the taking on board of medical advice takes an expected form, there is also activated a strong sense in which responsibility, independence, and proactive help-seeking is present. This was not an isolated incident—others in the sample also operated this 'double check'. For example, Basanti talked about her husband's diabetes, but in this case, it was an inverted check—the diagnosis took place in India during a holiday, and contrasted with a diagnosis by their GP in the UK:

The doctors knew nothing about this. He'd had some heart operations, then, we went to India, and he had some problems there, diarrhoea etc., and because he'd already had heart problems, we admitted him to hospital… and there, on the spot, blood tests and everything, and they asked if he was diabetic, we said no. They told us he has high levels of sugar in his blood. He wrote a letter to bring back to the GP. We went to see our doctor here and told him. He (the GP) said this can't be. He got tested, and then, it was confirmed.

Embedded in people's social activities are active conceptualisations of what the illness is, what action to take when a diagnosis is revealed, and how to activate a series of resources in order to optimise health status and illness management. While these socialities are, of course, mediated by any number of intersectional possibilities, related to age, gender, ethnicity, faith, and material position, the participants in this sample, being twice migrants (Bachu 1985), utilised their diasporic positions to mobilise agency in their medical encounters.

Familiarity or 'There's a Lot of It in Our Community!'

As a result of such high incidence and prevalence on a global basis, there is a sense in which this problem, while certainly not welcomed, may be partially expected. Many of the respondents were aware of the growing problem (it is often simply called a 'sugar problem'), and much of this familiarity came through families and social connections. Such 'knowing' is a common feature of those groups who have been predefined through science as 'high risk' (genetically or otherwise). For example, within the Pima Indian community of Arizona in Smith-Morris's ethnography (2006), there is an extensive, common, and detailed knowledge base about the many varied lifestyle, cultural, diet, and genetic risks which they are discursively embedded within. However, in Smith-Morris's study, the knowledge and awareness came as much from the long-established clinical research programmes in the area as from experiencing the illness themselves. Thus, social actors are exposed to, subjected to, and embroiled in many different health messages and enterprises as they go about their daily lives, and become, in one form or another, knowledgeable about the illness, especially in terms of the connection to their 'own' community.

Having someone in the immediate or extended family with diabetes functioned as an awareness-increasing tool regarding the general nature of the illness, the medication regimes, the required changes in lifestyle, and the physical effects. Familiarity also functioned as a buffer to reduce the emotional and psychological impact of the diagnosis. For example, Kanti, an 88-year-old woman explained:

> I didn't think anything (of the illness) because my mother had diabetes at the age of 30; well, I got it very late, and the doctor said it's not an inherited thing, it's because your pancreas is not working.

'*Apra ma bho che*' is a phrase used repeatedly in the interviews, and translates to 'there is a lot of it in our community'. The 'it' being referred to is 'sugar' or 'sugar diabetes'; to have 'sugar' or a 'sugar problem', therefore, is to have diabetes. In this sense, there was certainly a strong familiarity with the illness. When I initially explained the purpose and aims of the research, there was a general 'knowing-ness'—indicating the interview was characterised by a knowledge and familiarity of diabetes with specific reference to membership of an ethnically distinct group. When I asked participants about their first thoughts on knowing they had the condition, there were a variety of responses—some people did not report being overly anxious because of the experience and familiarity they already had, while for others, the same sense of familiarity was the cause for anxiety:

> Because my elder brother had it, and I saw his symptoms, as soon as I started having those symptoms, within a month, I went to see the doctor… when it came to my turn, I thought that's not right, so I went to the doctor. (Kishore, 59)
>
> At the time, I thought this is a dangerous thing, it can make you blind, heart problems, can give you lots of problems. So, you have to be very careful. I know one man who went blind. (Naresh, 72)

The idea of being familiar with the illness is important here because it illustrates that within groups of people, loosely defined as cultural communities, there is a level of knowledge about diabetes, which provides the basis for further exploration. This knowledge can be interpreted as 'lay health' beliefs, which have their own logic and consistency (Gerhardt 1987). However, they may also be thought of as 'access points', used by people to start the process of diabetes management. To have this familiarity often lessened the anxiety involved in the illness, but also served as a membership tool—hence the common phrase, *there's a lot of it in our community*. While the membership was not always welcomed—illness seldom is—respondents gained some source of comfort and support from there being a shared and collective illness space. This seemed to serve a useful purpose in terms of group membership and facilitated support and the active management of the illness. In a sense, participants could be seen as social actors taking on board health discourse information about 'South Asian diabetes' trends, but rather than passively accepting these constructions, they could be seen to be utilising them to manage their condition. In other words, they were articulating in lay terms what they understood to be happening in 'their community', and rather than fatalistically accepting this, they retained agency and control over their conditions. There is a general consensus (see Davies et al. 2009) regarding the way South Asian people view their diagnosis as inevitable and as something meant to be accepted with resignation mainly because of a family history of diabetes. Here, however, participants blatantly resist these formulations of passivity by actively utilising this familiarity as a source of empowerment.

Maclean (1991) discusses wisdom gained from experience and Kelleher (1988) discusses how this experience was sometimes more valuable in its specificity than a doctor's general knowledge. Here, however, familiarity does not need to stop at the persons' own experience of the illness and the body, but could certainly be extended to other people in the family or social circle with similar experiences. Additionally, this type of reflexive knowledge is not necessarily limited to adherence to diet, but could also be employed in what Reed (2003) identified as the transcultural and transglobal transferral of knowledge and remedies. The late or high Modern era is identified as being particularly individualistic, self-reflexive, and risk-laden (Giddens 1991). However, it is also an age of extensive globalisation, with technological and scientific frontiers being pushed to the limits of exploration mainly through the needs of mass communication and financial market operation. These technologies bring their own adaptational possibilities for accessing information, establishing diasporic connections between individuals and group who can be linked despite time and space limitations. Certainly, for many of the participants, their condition was not solely a feature of a one-dimensional route between self and expert systems. Rather, it was a single health issue which was one of many possibilities within a complex informational and identity network—especially if we recall that diabetes was already a 'community' issue they were aware of. Acquiring an official diabetes diagnosis was, of course, required and carried legitimacy, in much the same way as reported in other studies (e.g. Reed 2003). However, the diagnosis was often one of several trajectories for the health and illness state to be pursued, and as people tend to demonstrate in their everyday lives, actions/reactions are far from simplistic and not identifiable as contained within a 'cultural' or 'ethnic' marker.

'Exercise' and Activity

As part of both the general health education and health promotion literature surrounding illnesses such as diabetes, and other conditions (obesity, cardiovascular diseases, and depression), exercise has been noted as extremely important in the overall prevention and management of diabetes. Often, this has been in the form of prescriptive notions of specific amounts of physical activity for the general population; at other times, this has been targeted at specific groups, such as South Asians (e.g. Ramachandran et al. 2013). Participants seemed to be aware of a general health message regarding physical activity and diabetes, and that they, as a targeted 'high risk' group, had a responsibility to undertake this activity. There was also a sense in which they presented an admission of culpability—they did not exercise as much as they knew they should, and this contributed in some way to diabetes onset. However, there were also variously articulated counter-narratives and although people did reproduce generalised health messages about lack of exercise in their talk, they also went on to elaborate how they did manage some form of activity.

This seeming contradiction highlighted how, on the one hand, people were aware of the 'high risk package' that existed and their role within this, but on the other hand, were also self-aware of the actual practices in their daily lives which contested these representations. These, of course, are not mutually exclusive, since we can all find examples of health information about our practices which we regard as fairly accurate, whilst simultaneously demonstrating contradictory actions. As Sriskantharajah (2007) found in a study of South Asian women's perceptions of exercise, the incorporation of activity into daily life was more important than the 'Western' notion of an organised and specific exercise routine. Rina, Dhansuk, and Kanti talk about the reasons for the perceived lack of exercise in the generic South Asian community, as well as reasons for being able to partake in activity:

They tend to lead sedentary lives, sit in front of the telly; we Hoover, we used to sit on the floor, we never had a washing machine for 20 years; people don't walk anywhere, they get in a car. Most families have got 2 cars; I'm the same. Exercise and lifestyle, that's where it is. (Rina, 40)

Taking plenty of exercise, whatever you can... rather than living a very sedentary life, eating too much, just sleeping, not doing anything, being lethargic, that's a sure sign that you are suffering. (Dhansuk, 54)

I'm very careful with my food, no sugar in tea etc., but in rice and carbohydrates, you do get some sugar, so...I exercise as well, cycling, but walking is difficult because of the climate, and I've some problems with balance. (Kanti, 88)

A number of participants also explained to me that they took part regularly in yoga sessions, and while this was not extensive in the sample, it was the means by which they learnt about and engaged in the exercise which prompted attention. Interestingly, yoga has, in the recent past, been a dominant force in the health and well-being arena, being offered in leisure centres and fitness gyms globally. These spaces are not primarily places where elder Asians might frequent, but through the expansion of global telecommunication networks, it is now a popular choice in the homes of South Asians in Britain: '...Asian yoga is huge in the UK—this guy has come over from India who's a yoga teacher and there's a whole phenomenon of Asian housewives up and down the country doing yoga in front of their TV at 7 o'clock every day' (Douglas 2006). While the local temple in two of the sites (which also typically serves as a community centre) ran exercise classes for the over-50s, an additional event is the televised satellite broadcast from India. In these cases, people were able to watch yoga sessions broadcast from India, and listen to various forms of health advice from a religious and/or spiritual representative within the privacy of their own homes:

They show people just how many problems can disappear...I tried this yoga; it's made so much difference. There are even doctors there, who are being helped...I wake up at 5, do the exercises, (it) makes a difference. (Basanti, 65)

The presence of medical doctors taking part in the sessions on yoga broadcasts provides a scientific legitimacy, thereby transforming what might be a 'private' practice into a perfectly acknowledgeable 'public' practice. Overtly, this may be through the physical and practical ease with which one can access television and watch or record a programme, so that one can practice the exercises. However, symbolically, there is also the underlying validation these activities are given by the religious and/or spiritual position of the expert or 'guru'. Further validation is given when, as Basanti says above, 'even doctors are there', showing that even those who are practitioners of the biomedical paradigm can be engaged in terms of complementary and traditional health methods.

Basanti has weaved the yoga sessions into her daily life, though it is closely connected to her adoption and adherence to herbal and traditional remedies for a variety of illnesses (discussed in Chap. 7). The relevant point here is that through a transnational conduit, using modern media, there is a facility to maintain symbolic and physical interaction with cultural and ethnic diasporic identities. The concept of 'transnational' identity (Ramji 2006) has been well-established in discussions of the various aspects of migrant experiences in Britain and elsewhere. As Ramji explains, 'Transnationals are individuals whose sense of identity crosses multiple borders' (2006: 646), and this relates to the many ways in which migrants do not situate themselves in a binary position in relation to their country of 'origin' and the destination or settlement country. Rather, they 'create active social fields between the two… [Which]… involves various forms of movement, communication and long distance participation' (Ramji 2006: 646). While the participants here were not explicitly talking about their 'home' as anything other than their present location, they mobilised 'imagined communities' (Anderson 1991) and networks of belonging outside of their immediate location. As such, and as I have referred to in this book, their identities are diasporic, and as people who may well be settled here for a number of decades, also utilise diasporic connections and imaginaries.

Though participants show that exercise may be a contentious issue as far as diabetes and South Asians are concerned, there exists resistance to the formal constructions, and this is played out in people's innovative activities. Participants were able to talk about the possible causes of diabetes, such as sedentary lifestyles, poor nutrition, and lifestyles, but also, then talk about the ways in which they were active in their personal and social lives combating these 'risks'. These strategies were not individualised decisions; rather, they were part of wider social relations—when people made a decision to go for a walk, there was inevitably a role to be played by a friend or neighbour:

> Well, I go walking around here; one round is 40 minutes. Now, I walk a little more slowly, maybe it takes 50 minutes, 1 hour. Before I used to have company, my friend used to walk with me, but since he died, it's gotten less; then I had an operation done. Now I'm starting again. (Harish, 74)

Activity and exercise as concepts are not to be seen as uni-dimensional units of analysis, which are found in Western concepts of body health and fitness management. Rather, as people have expressed in this research, activity is more an expression of social and cultural management. Much in the same way that the modern Western, scientific idea and formal study of nutrition requires a 're-socialising' (Schubert et al. 2012), so the binaried bounding of 'physical' activity as either conforming to legitimate prescriptions of defined and measurable activity or illegitimate and deviant non-definable activities needs reconfiguring. Certainly, the widely recapitulated view that particular sets of norms, especially, for example, applied to groups of South Asian women are a serious barrier for both appropriate nutrition and activity (Davies et al. 2009) might need to be tempered with sociological and anthropological research. Such development might allow analysis of these contingent social entities to move away from the narrow confines of conceptually hegemonic and exclusionary notions of 'lifestyle' and exercise.

The Social and Cultural Context of Nutrition and Diabetes

Diet and nutrition have also been the focus of much discussion and research in South Asian health discourse. Many of the usual typological categories that are evoked are unhealthy and saturated fat diets, inappropriate cooking methods, lack of necessary vitamins and minerals (all of which have now been questioned), and these are invoked in the respondents' talk:

> You know the problem is that in our cooking, there's so much frying going on, that all the vitamins are gone. Boiling is the best, but oil ruins it. (Naresh, 72)
>
> In our communities, there's too much oil in the food, whereas in English cooking, its more boiled food, ours is oily. (Pramod, 59)
>
> They just don't look after themselves, they sit and have buttered cobs and samosas day in, day out. We've usually eaten by 7 pm, latest. People eat so late and go straight to bed; it's not good for them. (Rina, 40)

The negotiation of health status within a network of other dimensions of identity is a complex, but endlessly accomplished social, cultural, and personal activity. Within the narratives of people in this study, membership was accounted for by reference to cultural, ethnic, linguistic, migratory, and local groups, as well as 'imagined moral communities' (Chatoo and Ahmad 2004: 19; Seale 1998: 30). Naresh and Pramod are men in their late 50s and early 70s, respectively, and include themselves in the groups that may not cook in the healthiest way. Rina, however, who is of a younger generation (she is 40), a working professional, and involved in work within the South Asian community, uses the 'they' category. This may be a generalisation on her part, but she is morally accounting for practices in the community, and placing herself outside of this group. Similarly, here, Basanti and Kanti ensure I know about their 'healthy' practices:

> In my family's history we don't eat anything from outside. Since coming here in…my mum came here 1968, there were so many problems in getting our food, and yet, my family has never eaten frozen or tinned food. Always fresh. (Basanti, 65)
>
> I eat less now—I don't eat to a full stomach anymore; if I want 2 chapattis, I eat one and half; if I'm hungry for one and half, then I'll eat one. But I'll eat my curries, because that's where I get my greens, for stamina. (Kanti, 88)

Basanti above, a staunch advocate of natural and vegetarian food, who cooks for her immediate and extended family—as they live in a household with son, daughter-in-law, and grandchildren—takes pride in not having eaten processed or pre-prepared food. Kanti, meanwhile, tells me about how she is able to moderate her intake in a specialised way. There is differential calorific value applied to eating flour-based items such as chapattis, and eating fibre-laden green vegetables. Within these routine and mundane life routines, people talked about the many ways in which they attach importance to managing the many aspects of the condition, but do so in embedded social forms, not specifically separate, medicalised ones (or epidemiological ones). Given the fundamentally social, political, and cultural nature of eating and nutrition (Murcott 2002), it is not surprising that participants demonstrably showed this social action in public as well as private arenas. Certainly, it pays analytical and conceptual dividends to avoid using unitary socio-economic categories to order health and nutrition problems in various populations. This is especially the case since, as the participants here show, ethnic and cultural identity, belonging and biography can proffer multiple mediating and protective health possibilities, reflecting, as Garro and Lang state, 'Food and food pathways constitute complex codes for social relations and symbols of cultural identity and change' (1993: 322).

Resolving Everyday Conflicts: Food and Social Eating

The conceptualisation, preparation, and consumption of food are, of course, cultural and social entities mediated by both tradition and modernity (Bradby 1997). This means that how people think of and consume food—especially when there are added elements of the effects on their body and the social impact on their interactions—will be facilitated by ideas of 'social' eating and notions of moderation. In essence, the people here did not simply make—or indeed, not make—food decisions in a vacuum. Rather, they took on board the requirements of their physical body, and located them within a social and cultural space, acknowledging

that doing so would have impacts for their social and community relations. What people do regarding food intake when in a social situation
presents a particular issue for people with diabetes. Since type 2 diabetics
are required to manage and control their insulin levels through a combination of medication and diet, this presents a particular challenge. People
were quite pragmatic about what they did about these situations where
taking part in the food consumption ritual conflicted with their health
requirements:

> I just tell them I won't eat that, forget it. Because the temptation is always
> going to be there, but you have to think about yourself, and if I do eat this,
> then I'm the one who will suffer. (Naresh, 72)
>
> When its sweet stuff, especially if it's the blessing at the temple, then I'll
> have a bit, but a little. I won't lie (to you), It's not going to hurt you, but if
> you're eating this all the time, then that's different. (Sunita, 70)
>
> At Diwali, if you've gone somewhere and someone hands you sweet
> offerings, I won't have a whole bit, I'll have a little bit, and then no-one
> feels like I didn't; I won't feel I like I didn't either. Why do I need to tell
> them? I'm not ashamed of it.... If I need to tell people, I tell people, if they
> don't need to know, then they don't need to know. (Rina, 40)

The function of moderation mediated by social context can be dietary-
related, social etiquette-related, and/or stigma-related—all interconnect-
ing with diabetes. The relative impact of the disclosure of conditions is
mediated by the severity, length of time with the condition, and individual circumstances of the person. However, with diabetes, given the
condition's prominence in health media exposure, and the national dissemination of medical guidance and advice according to government policy, there is, it seems, little stigma attached to being known as someone
with diabetes. With the raised profile and awareness in various minority groups as well as on a general national level, diabetes has become
somewhat normalised, and with it, the range of prescribed management
activities have also become part of the positive lexicon. These movements
are in no small way attributed to both non-government agencies as well
as government health interventions, and often, the two are overlapping
and interconnected. Campbell et al. (2003) show through Kelleher's early

research (1988) that coping and normalisation play central roles in the agentive management of diabetes. Such normality in embodied medical experience when intersected by other dimensions of identity, such as race/ethnicity, age, gender, and class allows us to raise interesting questions about how people 'do' the personal and interactional work of 'normal' and 'routine' diabetes. Rather than an 'ethnically' specific idea, it is more a demonstration that people moderate their calorific intake and that these are always being played out against a social, cultural, and biographical backdrop. Through people's talk and interaction, it appears that their actions in both individual and social settings are expressive of non-passivity. Quite contrary to not only diabetes-specific health discourse in academic research and government research, but also participants' reports themselves of other South Asians, they indicate how the risk is demonstrably resisted and mitigated in everyday situations. They assess, monitor, and evaluate the weight of the social significance of eating against the effect it will have on their diabetes. As participants explained, at times, the reason for partaking is to avoid offending the host; at other times, it may have religious meaning, as in Sunita's situation. For her, a blessing from the temple is an absolute 'must', which has to be eaten in however little a portion one is limited to. Religion, for her, has played a central role in facilitating her management of not just diabetes but a range of adversities in life, and as other research corroborates, both organised religion and personal faith can play important roles in health promotion and recovery (Grace et al. 2008; Morjaria-Keval and Keval 2015). This moderation is integral to the nature of diabetes management, and certainly, in conditions such as type 1 diabetes, where insulin injections as well as dietary regulation are required, it is even more important. The physiological nature of type 2 diabetes lends itself to be within a constellation of social contexts, and so, we can begin to understand both the challenges and difficulties faced by interested health bodies, as well as some of the particular directions taken in dealing with the 'problem'. The question often conceptualised in research is 'how do we get (these) people to eat healthier?' and is certainly one which resonates in a general fashion across the whole of nutrition science. The question which might feasibly lead to more nuanced information is perhaps, 'what is it people are already doing which indicates multiple and complex management of not only food intake, but the entire social and material context in which that food consumption sits?' The existing network of practices in everyday life in diabetes management is maintained partly through nutritional balance. Kishore has called his moderation 'balancing your books'—a metaphor he uses in the interview to explain to me how he conceptualises the management of the illness:

> Take today, I'm going to have a meal, and have a sweet offering, but I'll make sure I won't have anything else. I'm going to balance my books; I'll use it wisely here. For us diabetics, if you don't eat that sweet, then you have the option to eat 5 or 6 different items. In the ladvu (sweet desert), it is solid and packed with sugar and you've spent your money. Whereas the other way, there's curry, salad, this, that, you can spend it wisely. (Kishore, 59)

He goes onto to tell me that this 'balancing one's books' is how he explains diabetes management to other people that he meets in the community. It is a financial accounting metaphor, and one which he finds useful to implement and communicate, given his own training and background (accountancy). He finds this an easy method to relate the calorific intake management for diabetics on a day-to-day basis. For example, he enthuses about another of his metaphors:

> You control your diabetes manually—it's not an automatic car, with one of those all you have to do is operate the brake, when its manual you have to make sure you change the gears all the time; diabetes is like that. The sugar control is manual.

What is evidenced above is again the life-embedded nature of everyday health negotiation that people in this sample demonstrated. None of them were officially recognised, trained, or certified as skilled or professional in any way connected to diabetes (except for Dhansuk, who had fulfilled the requirements of the government's Expert Patient Programme). This was derived from connecting with life experiences and biographical backgrounds in order to manage the condition, and also communicate advice to other people.

Conclusion

The superficially straightforward idea of being diagnosed is here revealed to be both mundane and complex, often revealed by a chance occurrence and is mediated by and through culturally located ideas, but also connections that are wider than the individual's immediate space. Connections in India and other countries allowed for a buffer zone of acceptance, and as Naresh and Basanti explained above, sometimes, the diagnosis would not simply be accepted, and a differential system would be utilised. Not all the respondents had the facility or opportunity to do this, of course, as this required confidence and connections overseas, even if these connections would just send a newspaper article or were available over the telephone. However, far from being isolated or deviant cases, they represent different forms of a common thread. Even those respondents who did not have overseas connections were able to employ proactive systems in the diagnosis process, negotiating diet and nutrition, and taking part in exercise. Many of these systems were related to religious beliefs, but some were also active social networks and the biographical accumulation of experiences of adversity which, as migrants to the UK with an array of life experiences, these participants held to be important. Proactivity mediated by familiarity, social networks, and in some cases, religious frameworks reinforced the individual's ability to cope with the condition. Even though there was talk of culpability and blame—sometimes allocated to 'people in our community', sometimes to themselves, it was the private, personal body, as embedded within social and cultural contexts that was the site of activity, and therefore, the site of counter-high-risk narratives. These emerged in ways which, although show uncertainties, disruptions, and changes in people's lives, also show demonstrable notions of continuity. Using aspects of their cultural identity, and their biographies, histories, and experiences, counter-narratives emerged, which resisted the high-risk constructions I have been discussing. Through this resistance, people here were creating and maintaining personal and social order, negotiating relationships with family and other networks, and weighing up the impacts on social connections. They used knowledge of their own bodies and the relation to external structures to negotiate how diabetes was positioned in their lives. In the following chapter, I explore through these counter-narratives how people in this group used a variety of different health remedies as part of their health negotiations.

References

Ahmad, W. I. U., & Bradby, H. (2007). Locating ethnicity and health: Exploring concepts and contexts. *Sociology of Health & Illness, 29*(6), 795–810. Available at: http://www.ncbi.nlm.nih.gov/pubmed/17986016. Accessed 13 Nov 2014.

Anderson, B. (1991). *Imagined communities: Reflections on the spread of nationalism*. London: Verso.

Bachu, P. (1985). *Twice migrants*. London: Tavistock.

Bradby, H. (1997). Health, eating and heart attacks: Glaswegian Punjabi women's thinking about everyday food. In *Food, health and identity*. London: Routledge.

Brah, A. (2006). The Asian in Britain. In N. Ali, V. S. Kalra, & S. Sayyid (Eds.), *A postcolonial people – South Asians in Britain* (pp. 35–61). London: Hurst and Company.

Bulmer, M. (1987). *The social basis of community care*. London: Allen and Unwin.

Campbell, R., et al. (2003). Evaluating meta-ethnography: A synthesis of qualitative research on lay experiences of diabetes and diabetes care. *Social Science and Medicine, 56*(4), 671–684. Available at: http://www.sciencedirect.com/science/article/pii/S0277953602000643. Accessed 18 Nov 2014.

Chattoo, S., & Ahmad, W. I. U. (2004). The meaning of cancer: Illness, biography and social identity. In D. Kelleher & G. Leavey (Eds.), *Identity and health* (pp. 19–36). London: Routledge.

Cornwell, J. (1984). *Hard earned lives: Accounts of health and illness from East London*. London: Tavistock.

Davies, M. J., Yates, T., & Khunti, K. (2009). Prevention of type 2 diabetes. In K. Khunti, S. Kumar, & J. Brodie (Eds.), *Diabetes UK and South Asian Health Foundation recommendations on diabetes research priorities for British South Asians*. London: Diabetes UK.

Diabetes UK. (2013). State of the nation – England. Available at: http://www.diabetes.org.uk/Documents/About%20Us/What%20we%20say/0160b-state-nation-2013-england-1213.pdf. Accessed 2 Jul 2014.

Douglas, T. (2006, August 16). A Muslim 'digital ghetto'? *BBC News*, Vol. 15, p. 27. http://news.bbc.co.uk/1/hi/uk/4798813.stm

Fee, M. (2006). Racializing narratives: Obesity, diabetes and the 'aboriginal' thrifty genotype. *Social Science and Medicine, 62*, 2988–2997.

Ferreira, M., & Lang, G. (2006). *Indigenous peoples and diabetes: Community empowerment and wellness.* Durham: Carolina Academic Press.

Garro, L. C., & Lang, G. C. (1993). Explanations of diabetes: Anishinaabeg and Dakota deliberate upon a new illness. In J. R. Joe & R. S. Young (Eds.), *Diabetes as a disease of civilisation: The impact of culture change on indigenous peoples.* New York: Mouton de Gruyter.

Gerhardt, U. (1987). Parsons, role theory and health interaction. In G. Scambler (Ed.), *Sociological theory and medical sociology.* London: Tavistock.

Giddens, A. (1991). *Modernity and self-identity.* Cambridge: Polity Press.

Grace, C., Begum, R., Subhani, S., Kopelman, P., & Greenhalgh, T. (2008). Prevention of type 2 diabetes in British Bangladeshis: Qualitative study of community, religious, and professional perspectives. *BMJ, 337*, a1931. doi:10.1136/bmj.a1931.

Gupta, S., de Belder, A., & O'Hughes, L. (1995). Avoiding premature coronary deaths in Asians in Britain: Spend now on prevention or pay later for treatment. *British Medical Journal, 311*, 1035–1036.

Helman, C. G. (1990). Culture, health and illness. Available at: http://www. sciencedirect.com/science/article/pii/B9780723619918500085

Hill, J. (2006). Management of diabetes in South Asian communities in the UK. *Nursing Standard, 20*(25), 57–64.

International Diabetes Federation. (2013). *IDF diabetes atlas* (6th ed.). Brussels: International Diabetes Federation. Available at: http://idf.org/diabetesatlas/download-book. Accessed 2 Jul 2014.

Kelleher, D. (1988). *Diabetes.* London: Routledge.

Lawton, J., Peel, E., Parry, O., Araoza, G., & Douglas, M. (2005). Lay perceptions of type 2 diabetes in Scotland: Bringing health services back in. *Social Science & Medicine, 60*, 1423–1435.

Maclean, H. M. (1991). Patterns of diet related self-care in diabetes. *Social Science and Medicine, 32*(6), 689–696.

Mechanic, D. (1978). *Medical sociology.* New York: Free Press.

Morjaria-Keval, A., & Keval, H. (2015). Reconstructing Sikh spirituality in recovery from alcohol addiction. *Religions, 6*(1), 122–138.

Murcott, A. (2002). Nutrition and inequalities: A note on sociological approaches. *The European Journal of Public Health, 12*(3), 203–207. Available at: http://eurpub.oupjournals.org/cgi/doi/10.1093/eurpub/12.3.203.

Nazroo, J. (1997). *The health of Britain's ethnic minorities: Findings from a national survey*. London: Policy Studies Institute.

Parekh, B. (2007). Reasoned identities: A committed relationship. In M. Wetherall, M. LaFleche, & R. Berkeley (Eds.), *Identity, ethnic diversity and community cohesion*. London: Sage.

Qureshi, B. (1989). *Transcultural medicine*. Dordrecht: Kluwer.

Ramachandran A, Snehalatha C, Samith Shetty A, Nanditha A. (2013). Primary prevention of Type 2 diabetes in South Asians--challenges and the way forward. *Diabet Med. Jan;30*(1):26-34. doi: 10.1111/j.1464-5491.2012. 03753.x.

Ramji, H. (2006). British Indians 'returning home': An exploration of transnational belongings. *Sociology, 40*(4), 645–662.

Reed, K. (2003). *Worlds of health: Exploring the health choices of British Asian mothers*. London: Praeger.

Rock, M. (2005). Figuring out type 2 diabetes through genetic research: Reckoning kinship and the origins of sickness. *Anthropology & Medicine, 12*(2), 115–127.

Schubert, L., Gallegos, D., Foley, W., & Harrison, C. (2012). Re-imagining the 'social' in the nutrition sciences. *Public Health Nutrition, 15*(2), 352–359. Available at: http://www.ncbi.nlm.nih.gov/pubmed/21729468. Accessed 13 Nov 2014.

Seale, C. (1998). *Constructing death*. Cambridge: Cambridge University Press.

Smith- Morris, C. (2006). *Diabetes among the Pima: Stories of survival*. Tucson: University of Arizona Press.

7

Using Complementary Health and Remedies

Introduction

So far, I have asserted that in a discussion of the health–ethnicity relationship, it is important to be able to conceptualise the historical and contemporary terms of engagement with the area, but also to think critically about the nature of difference, and how it is dealt with over time. How a specific polity in a given time period deals with minority populations is reflected in how the same minority populations may experience health and illness. Intersecting this narrative arc is the condition of diabetes, and its biomedical, physiological, and treatment-led character. As with most health-related issues, the nature of help-seeking for diabetes is neither straightforward nor simplistic, and features a number of context-providing glimpses into the socio-cultural, diasporic, and biographical aspects. The use of healthcare from multiple sources and providers is also indicative of the use of a wide ranging set of personal, cultural, and social resources, themselves mediated by both local and global networks of belonging. What we find here in the study of diabetes is that participants were using a variety of different systems of health and help for both their specific condition and their general well-being, and that these ideas were

© The Editor(s) (if applicable) and The Author(s) 2016
H. Keval, *Health, Ethnicity and Diabetes*,
DOI 10.1057/978-1-137-45703-5_7

sourced in their social, ethnic, cultural, migrational, and biographical identities. Participants in this study talked about their use of a range of overlapping and connected healthcare remedies—from visits to the GP and 'official' medication, traditional herbal and folk remedies which they already knew of or had gleaned information about through networks, through to a narrative reconnecting with past experiences and biographical accounts of personal histories. What is important, as Reed (2003) argues is that people have membership of lots of different, connected local and global networks, and that both products and services are utilised in a reflective way to assess the 'fit' with whatever their current 'official' allopathic care system advocates. Such use, then, is interconnected with a variety of cultural and ethnic, migrational aspects that show how people utilise frameworks for living, and negotiating the complex arena of seeking help.

Using Traditional and Herbal Remedies

The use of traditional medicines for a variety of illnesses is not a new phenomenon in the South Asian community or on a global basis. Herbal medicines have been quoted in use since 6000 BC (in the ancient Hindu texts Rig Veda and Ayurveda), with 600 plant species being used in various formulations (Subbulakshmi and Naik 2001). An estimated 80 % of people living in (so-called) 'less developed' countries rely exclusively on traditional medicine (Farnsworth 1988). The use of complementary and alternative medicine has been widely treated in both research and practice (Cant and Sharma 2003), and is an area of great diversity and divergence in how it is conceptualised. Although there are a number of studies which examine the use of these complementary remedies (e.g. Bhopal 1986; Wood et al. 2004), they have not traditionally been the focus of much of the literature within the field. An important aspect of this discussion lies in how these traditional systems are situated in social imaginaries. By this, I refer to the view that these systems cannot be viewed as simply compartments of knowledge, there to be used or ignored in isolation, but rather, as indicative of both historical and contemporary markers of identity. As Ahmad (1993: 28) points out in his critique of the racial politics of health, 'colonisation' processes extend beyond territories and people, to knowledge, cultures, and values. Therefore, traditional forms of knowledge such as Ayurveda, certainly in India and other parts of South Asia, were discredited and discursively identified as non-effective, and outside of mainstream science. This historical context to 'Western' medical hegemony is important here to bear in mind since the participants are part of the colonial and postcolonial fabric of British cultural makeup, and with their migration histories, they brought biographical remnants of multiple systems of knowledge. Knowing about traditional medicines and herbal remedies was not simply about 'lay knowledge', but an accomplishment of cultural maintenance and reproduction. To know that certain roots and herbs have specific effects on the various bodily mechanisms and operations, which could contribute to better diabetes management, was a system of skill and knowledge passed inter-generationally and internationally. This global and local health positioning may be characterised by 'lay' knowledge, but is, more fundamentally, a demonstration of culturally located health and illness management through personal biographical and social resources.

Reorienting 'Other' Systems of Health

Established discussions of complementary and alternative medicine (CAM) systems focus on changes in the relationship between practitioner groups and the state (Cant and Sharma 2003) so that what is being underlined is professional and political comparisons between official groups. The use of herbal remedies—while certainly having overlaps with officially recognised and established CAM systems such as Ayurveda— do not reflect an official, expert system. Rather, there is a difference between an official and 'expert system' of medical training and what can be classed here as the anthropologically informed ethno-medicine, or the 'folk' component of Kleinmans' (1988) popular, professional, and folk triad, which sits comfortably as an alternative element within the range of extant healing pluralities. The terminology is also important, as Saks (1992) argues that a term such as 'complementary medicine' can conflict with the fundamental bases between types of medicine. He suggests the term 'alternative' because it more readily takes into account the division between those ideas supported by the medical establishment, and those which are not. The naming process, as Gale (2014) shows, is an exercise in power, since the notions of complementary and alternative are both loaded with symbolic meanings, themselves pointing to central and periphery, core and marginalised systems. There is much discussion of the notion of 'medical pluralism'—the complex network of transactions between institutions and individuals (Comelles et al. 2007), professionalisation, and questions about efficacy in relation to the state of CAM. Much of the established research and discourse in CAM is rooted in the provision of what might be termed 'alternative' services, and the extent and nature of people's usage of these services. There are a number of central components which can feasibly help us to make sense of the importance of these help-seeking trajectories in light of the book's central aim—to unpack the discursive constructions of passivity and high risk of South Asian populations.

Again, these are debates of profession and politics, and by and large, do not represent what people were actually doing or practising in their private lives. However, it does open up the issue of where 'folk' or 'lay' medicine can be placed comfortably, especially those which are situated in 'local knowledges' and biographical, experiential histories. While the disadvantages of using some herbal remedies have been documented (Wood et al. 2004), the participants in this study were quite aware of the advantages and disadvantages of their usage—albeit not necessarily biomedical or biochemical awareness. The important feature is that these herbs were used with medical systems, and even then, it seems only when there was a background knowledge of the product. Once any adverse side effects were felt, the usage was stopped, and in some cases, there was a strong scientific case made by the participant for the need for control in these usages because of the unknown nature of the active compound. It came as little surprise that participants in this study had knowledge of these remedies, and in many cases, used them extensively. However, what is interesting and relevant is how these remedies are used, the ways in which both the physical and intellectual products are acquired, and how we can interpret both their usage and what people say about them.

Resituating Knowledge Through Experience: Using Tradition

Participants talked about a range of non-allopathic remedies, some of which were commonly used as herbs and spices in cooking, such as *methi* (fenugreek), *harddar* (turmeric), and *ajmo* (ajwain), while others were vegetables such as *karela* (bitter gourd), which were widely known and used as a remedy for diabetes. Other less well-known items were also mentioned, such as a 'root' substance and a general 'bitter' powder, which people ingest to help control glucose levels in the body. There was also a variety of ways in which these items were taken—from powdered forms taken with water, cooked as a curry or snacks, as a liquid form, and even crushed skins of the vegetable 'karela' turned into ice cubes. Some participants required prompting and specific questioning about their use of 'any other' remedies or medicines, while others, such as Deena, (aged 70) decided to talk about these complementary remedies very soon into the interview and talked openly:

> I always check my levels, and then take my tablets, and if I need to, I'll have some chocolate or something. I'll also take some 'kurvat ni phaki' …this makes quite a difference to me. This is from Dubai—I take just a little sometimes in the night when I wake up…whatever happens I always take my medication, but then if things get bad, I take a carefully measured amount and take that as well…I use karela as well, I use this quite often…I make a curry out of this and Methi, and I make steamed Methi—I've made some today.

When I ask Deena about her glucose levels, she tells me about how she checks it, and the herb she takes, including where it is from:

> Yes I do, I check sugar, 2–3 times in a week. If I feel my head has become heavy, then I check. Sometimes if it's too low or too high at night, I check. If it's too low, then I'll have a chocolate or something. If it's too high, then I'll take a tablet or have some bitters… it really makes a difference.

She goes on to tell me when she takes it, and importantly, that it is used as a complement to the prescribed tablets, not an alternative:

Often, when I wake up, then I take it first thing, 3, 4, 5 am, then I take a little with water, 2 glasses of water. I always take tablets as prescribed, but after that, I'll take this if I need to.

Rajesh (aged 51) tells me that this combining of remedies, this 'syncrecy', is effective for him:

I do take herbal. Somebody sent them from India, one tablet per day. I've been taking this remedy since the last 6–8 months… I mean, my results were around 7, since I started that remedy—plus my normal medication.

In the above extract, we are being informed that 'efficacy' is reached through the use of a herbal tablet—sourced from India, which is common in this sample—and the assessment of this efficacy is in purely medical terms—the participant's 'Hb' levels (HbA1c is a test that measures the amount of glycosylated haemoglobin in blood and provides a good estimate of how well diabetes is being managed over time). He is comfortable in expressing his blood sugar level in scientific/medical terms as used in much professional diabetes literature and education, but is equally comfortable in invoking different knowledge systems. This 'syncretic' approach is a common practice for the people in this study and symbolises the variety of connections participants had to different areas of traditional and contemporary healing ideas. Additionally, it symbolises social action manifested as a form of counter-narrative to constructions of passive health and/or a risk-laden South Asian diabetic identity. I do not argue that participants themselves consciously and explicitly formulate political activism (though it does not exclude this possibility) through these choices. Rather, their talk and action about the micro negotiations of diabetes and health in daily life can be interpreted as a form of *embodied resistance*, in much the same way that recent medical anthropological work (e.g. Ferreira and Lang 2006) identifies and participates in amplifying hitherto silenced and marginalised voices.

In a sense, we can seek to explore and excavate those things that people do and involve themselves in, which point to forms of contestation of hegemonic discursive practices. As Johnston (2002) cogently reminds us (in the context of Native American community relations), such usage of folk, herbal remedies—termed indigenous—serves as a conduit for people to express identities, not in a vacuum, but rather, in relation to overarching histories and struggles with dominant social structures. The research here does not purport to explore the various long and hard struggles that migrant communities have endured, but does assert that those complex experiences and biographies are part of the myriad expressions of help-seeking and negotiation. This type of medical or 'New' pluralism (Cant and Sharma 1999) or what Johnston views as 'apolitical pluralism' (2002) can find an important purchase in the lives and daily imaginings of South Asian people with diabetes in ways not attended to explicitly or consistently by dominant diabetes and health discourses. Gale (2014) conceptualises these activism possibilities as anti-hegemonic spaces in which culturally authorised biomedical power is challenged by the critique of 'integration'. In other words, if we conceptualise CAM, indigenous medicines, and folk remedies as being on the margins of 'real' medicine, then they are seen to require integration and become more like the dominant biomedical model. The parallels with how diversity and minority populations are handled and policed (discussed above) are clear, especially when we set this against the accepted normalisation of diabetes prevention and treatment regimes. Hence, we can view these ethno-folk help-seeking models as ways that help us make sense of the socialities inherent in people's help-seeking routes. Again, and as will be discussed below, there is both an international element in terms of sourcing the product and a local one, as many of the items mentioned here are widely available in South Asian grocery shops throughout the UK, as indicated in Naresh's excerpt:

> Oh yes, it's very good. I eat Methi in the morning, it's the best stuff. I make a powder out of it, in the morning I have it with some water… there's iron in it to help with strength and coping with pains. I've got to this age and yet I've never had hip problems. Then there's this 'Jambu' (Eugenia jambolana) powder, that's really the best for diabetes, which they sent us from India.

The variety of products people used was sourced locally and internationally, and used in combination with other products, including the prescribed medicines. The emphasis in many of these interviews was that there was a strict adherence to the prescribed medication for diabetes, but also, a parallel adherence to traditional and herbal remedies, which were part of a persons' cultural history, and maintained through local and international connections. The local–global dialectic (Giddens 1991) is an interesting sociological phenomenon, which utilises the post-traditional frame as a driving force for much of the relationship between reflexivity and health (Reed 2003). Such thinking through, and cognisance, about one's position in a risk-laden society, as Beck (1992) and others have explored, is part of the complex fabric of 'risk society', and involves the implication of an erosion of trust in 'expert systems' with an increasing sense and practice of 'choice'. These interpretations of fluidity, dynamicism, and agentive articulations of belonging, history, and culture to make sense of diabetes and health need to be set alongside and interwoven with any number of intersectional experiences of material position, race, gender, and age, for example. As Reed (2003) warns us, using ideas such as syncrecy can be revealing, but also, runs the risk of masking the enduring, entrenched, and real rather than imagined problems of intersectional inequalities. The differences between aspirations for and realities of postmodern utopias, where identities move between and beyond categorisation, have been critiqued elsewhere in detail (e.g. Cross and Keith 1992). In this section, I assert that the interpretation of folk and ethno medicine is principally to *highlight* rather than *mask* the dynamic negotiations of everyday 'risk' within a social and cultural landscape which is imbued with materiality. In line with this active negotiation of help-seeking for diabetes, there were many ideas participants had about why they might use herbal and/or traditional remedies. Some of the participants had heard about a 'diabetes-related' herb or vegetable from a friend or family member, and others talked about the family tradition of using these methods:

> Well, at the moment I'm eating 'Methi' (fenugreek)—you put it in water overnight and just drink the water…I'm just trying…because I do believe in Ayurvedic medicine. But I'm also very pro-western medicine as well—tablets and things like that, because I think they have put in a lot of research into it and a lot of effort and a lot of money, and come out with these sorts of tablets, so they must be good… it's a question of trial and error (Dhansuk, 54).

Echoing Rajesh's excerpt, Dhansuk's use, or in this case, his trying out of traditional medicines is perfectly combined with allopathic medicines and there is a dual recognition of scientific and traditional efficacy—similar to Basanti's statement regarding the presence of medical doctors appearing in yoga broadcasts from India providing scientific legitimacy. Kanti tells me what she takes as a remedy, but more importantly, why she takes it:

> Firstly, I take a quarter spoon turmeric, with warm water, then in another glass, a quarter spoon methi, and in a third glass, quarter spoon ajmo. So, in the stomach, the gas is lessened. As we get older, the digestion power is weakened, so food isn't digested as easily (Kanti, 88).

In the excerpt above, Kanti talks about herbs commonly found in most South Asian households as well as most grocery shops which stock South Asian cooking ingredients. These items are taken systematically as a routine, quite like a prescribed medication—but the reasoning behind their use is explained. There is an acknowledgement that the ageing process brings about weakness and gradual degradation of the body—which can be managed by using these herbs:

> Look, turmeric is an antibiotic. So I don't need to take antibiotics. Otherwise, a lot of the time for diabetics, they have to take this and that, but with me, where I have been hurt, it won't go infected; otherwise, usually if you get hurt, you have to take an antibiotic. I burnt myself about 5–6 months ago…now it would usually become infected, but with me, no, so the antibiotic is there, and Ajmo lessens gas and helps digestion.

The use of these herbs, however, is not just illness-specific—sometimes, it is a generalised belief in their efficacy, as told here by Basanti, who uses them extensively alongside allopathic prescriptions:

> Methi, linseed, my son takes a bottle with him, my grandchildren, all take it. Just at the weekend, I gave them all doses. At the moment, they've all got colds, so I put together a remedy—mixture, liquorice, turmeric, some others. It helps. When my grandchild was born, they said he had asthma—we used only these herbal remedies, and he's never needed the pump.

The generalised use of these remedies passes inter-generationally, and has both a routine and focused use. The implication for diabetes is that both Bikhu (58) and Basanti (65) (partners in marriage), who use allopathic and traditional remedies, are able to manage their illness, but also extend this use to their immediate family. The cultural tradition of herbal, traditional, or Ayurvedic systems is maintained inter-generationally, from a focused and illness-specific personal use, to a general health preventative use for grandchildren. Again, this demonstrates that participants such as Bikhu and Basanti did not show a polarised medicine use, nor was it binaried, as they used several forms in combination, even though they were clear about which system was better in the long run:

> The chemicals that go into medicine—in our 'desi' (Indian) medicine, there's nothing like that. Ok, the effects may take longer, it's more long-term, but it does make a difference.

The possibility of the side effects of allopathic medicines is also discussed by some participants, who were reassured by the naturalness of herbal remedies. When I asked about the combined use of diabetes medication and herbal remedies, Naresh replied, '*It's fine, there's no side effects to it, it's all herbal.*' Kanti was also acutely aware of the effects which biomedicine seemed to have on her, describing it as a 'Mahabharata' (a religious narrative about war, located in the history and mythology of Hinduism) in her body:

> Recently, I found the medicine has had reverse effects on my body—so I went to the doctor and I said I don't want any medicine apart from diabetes medicine. Herbal medicines haven't got reverse effects, these have. You know we say about Mahabharata, I said if it (biomedicine) goes into my body, there will be Mahabharata in my body. So, I don't want any war now. When I did not understand, I took it, but now I understand that it has given me reverse effects, I stopped it.

These demonstrations of the 'naturalness' of the herbs and vegetables people are using have also been observed by Sharma (1995), underlining the concern about the possible side effects of biomedicine.

The articulations of efficacy and safety are rooted in explanatory frameworks of both culture and ethnicity. There is a sense in many of these narratives of traditional, herbal remedies being firmly located both within a cultural and ethno-religious positioning, so that the knowledge of these remedies, as well as the ability to utilise them, comes from a Gujarati identity and a faith-related belonging (here, a Hindu identity). This is interesting because it helps to demonstrate how syncretic usage of systems is not usefully characterised as an 'either–or' binary unit, but rather, as a dialectical relationship. There are parallels here between the use of participants' knowledge of Ayurvedic humours and Western humoral formulations—the body's need to be in a balanced state consisting of 'hot' and 'cold' elements (Helman 1994). For example, as Helman tells us, English lay health beliefs about 'feeding a cold and starving a fever' stem from these ideas of counteraction (1994: 14). Humoral theory rests on the idea that all substances have a hot or cold element to them—a 'symbolic power' (Helman 1994: 13)—and for optimum health, the body must be in a balance between these two states. In Ayurvedic medicine, there is a complex interplay of the constituents and inter-constituents of basic elements of the universe and the body—health and illness rest on the interaction between them. The embodied 'balancing' act rests upon the homeostatic alignment between hot and cold elements (Ramakrishna and Weiss 1992). It is conceptually easier to render these as cultural, ethnic, and global differences as also echoing differences between perhaps industrialised modern nations, and reflecting beliefs still caught in the transformative process of global capitalism. However, the parallels and commonalities between systems are of interest, and are supported by Jobanputra's (2005) findings that there was no significant health belief difference between British Gujarati Indian immigrants and British White people. However, I intend not to make comparisons between groups—this runs the risk of setting up a conceptual system of 'other-ness', whereby health belief models and deficits in knowledge are assessed in relation to a group's ascribed cultural identity. Rather, there are sociological and anthropological commonalities in how lay and folk understandings of different types of health knowledge systems work together.

Situating Knowledge

Margaret Everett tells us, 'Illness is a vehicle for individual and cultural meaning, and that suffering expresses social and not merely biological events' (2011: 1781). Diabetes then becomes the vehicle for, first, understanding how health and illness are dynamically negotiated by South Asian people in the UK, but second, how these active socialities are forms of embodied social and cultural resistance to the prevailing racialised cultural and genetic discursive constructions of 'high risk'. Part of this picture is the willingness of participants in the research to talk about their histories, and they demonstrated a variety of ways in which health and illness are related to the social context of daily life, connected to history, biography, and experience. Many of the participants talked of specific experience, such as Kanti, who revealed she had begun training in medicine, before she was forced through family circumstances to abandon her studies:

> In India, my (school) principal was a European, and the science teaching was very good. It was one of the best state schools, the medium of instruction was English, so we don't have problems with this. From that, I decided to study medicine, first I got a sponsorship to study medicine, I did 2 years. As a teacher, I expanded my knowledge, in Nairobi, I was known as a doctor without certificate ... I know 'desi' medicine and other medicine.

This complementary and syncretic use of medical systems permeates many of the interviews in this study, and characterises in a useful way what Eade (1997) pinpointed as cultural construction. In this study, it also serves to demonstrate that a participant's notion of their position in the UK is not limited by time and place. Rather, it is fluid across histories, places, and the life course, pointing towards the overlap between diasporic and transnational identities (Ramji 2006). This fluidity is manifested in being familiar with different types of treatment and health conceptualisation. Deena, a widow, talked of how she knows about the remedies:

> Well, we're from India, and my mother and others used to use them. My brother was really very big on these remedies. Very often, he would write to me and tell me about them. Gas in the stomach, for example, my brother

would make up all these tablets and send them to me. So, I used them here as well…We know all this because we were in India. I came here after 40 years in India, I was a teacher there in school.

In using methi in her curries, Deena is employing a cultural framework, which takes local knowledge as its base. These 'knowledges', as Ferreira et al. (2006) have elucidated in recent medical anthropological studies, are part of the biographical and historical make-up of a group of people. How this knowledge is acquired, learned, and utilised symbolises very much the antithesis of 'passivity' and 'culturalist' explanations which have been put forward in the past in relation to this area. Using these herbs and vegetables and maintaining the practices which were learned as part of growing up can be regarded as a way of locating and maintaining one's sense of self and identity. Given that food and the rituals surrounding its preparations and sourcing, especially in light of ethno-medicine and 'folk remedies', has an important position in cultural and social contexts (Helman 1994), this can be seen as a biographical connection to place and time situated in healing and health practices. These connections are not asserted here as representative of some isolated and reified notion of 'ethnicity' or 'minority culture', but instead, as a form of cultural capital which, as Chacko says, gives us a sense of how 'preference for specific therapies is informed by the cultural heritage and natural environment…' (2003: 1088).

This sense in which participants were gradually telling a story not just about the ostensible 'diabetes research' nature of the work, but more accurately, about their life positions was present in most of the interview situations. This, however, is not to be located statically as a reified outcome of the research, but rather is inherently and intimately woven into the fabric of the relationship between the methodology employed here and the overall study. As Nettleton states, 'when people have the opportunity to give voice to their experience of illness, it becomes evident that their accounts are woven into their biographies' (2006: 81). Participants are compelled to involve their history and migration experiences in their explanations of how they have come to know the things they know. When they talk about how they know about herbal remedies for diabetes, they are maintaining a cultural connection in temporal, spatial, and symbolic orders. In other words, by using the 'illness narrative' (Kleinman 1988) as a mechanism for communicating biography, which is necessarily over a period of time and space, participants are able to get across a notion of their identity. The 'toolkit' or structures of relevance (Schutz 1966) used to make an informed decision about the use of herbal or Ayurvedic remedies are tied up with many contextual identity-related factors. In line with one of the main themes of this book, the cultural and ethnic identity of minority groups— in this case, South Asians—is neither a prescribed and allocated unity nor a completely self-maintained entity. The dialectical nature of ethnicity in this complex set of identities involves internal process as well as external forces (Nagel 1994). If we located this dialectical tension at the intersec- tion of 'medical pluralism' or folk and traditional healing and help-seeking, then we can observe how health and identity plays out in dynamic ways.

Conclusion

The use of different types of diabetes and general health remedies sourced from a variety of different knowledge bases, some in the biomedical model and some in traditional and folk remedies, indicates a number of possibilities. It demonstrates that far from the picture of 'cultural' pathol- ogy and passivity rendered by previous discourses of the last few decades, people in this study utilised the resources around them in a variety of dif- ferent ways, towards the twin goals of diabetes management and overall health status. Participants weave multiple aspects of their identity into negotiating health and illness. This multivocality of the experience as man- ifested in these 'lay health beliefs' prove to be strategic bridges in dealing with the management of illness and the management of the wider net- work of adversity. Some of these experiences are highlighted here in order to contextualise the diabetic experience. The context emphasises that the management of chronic conditions cannot be understood or investigated without necessarily problematising the nature of existing approaches and taking into account people's already existing skills. These skills or varieties of cultural capital lie in maintaining cultural and ethnic connections locally and internationally, through the use of different knowledge systems and help-seeking practices, while firmly adhering to the biomedical advice and medicines they have been prescribed. Participants ranged from knowing a great deal about the technical details of diabetes management and calorie intake effects on insulin and blood, to knowing very little of a technical nature. However, even those in the latter group were able to actively negotiate their help-seeking in the form of remedies through the use of various sources. It is important, as Eade (1997) argues, to demonstrate what these products and practices come to symbolise. They can point to a range of social, personal, and cultural processes concerning how, specifically, diabetes is conceptualised and managed, and more generally, health and illness states are attended to. Crucially, the additional facet of this is that it also provides a link between the individual and society—the agency structure question. Studies that look at the use of herbal practices—the intellectual product in the form of the knowledge as well as the physical relationship involved in getting hold of the products—are useful for rendering a picture of the pliability of individual and group processes working within wider social and structural constraints.

The use of these herbal remedies and specific health-enabling vegetables and products were embedded within personal and biographical frameworks, mediated by both individual and collective histories, which would be then the subject of public and social accounting during the interview. While individuals felt that these systems of knowledge were personal to themselves, they were also aware of these 'knowledges' (Worsley 1997) as membership markers, symbolising group membership to an ethnic, cultural, and biographical collectivity. The cultural negotiations demonstrated in the implementation of knowledge about different forms of remedy can be conceptualised as forms of embodied resistance to constructions of passive and pathologised cultural reification. This chapter situates one aspect of the type 2 diabetes experience within a social and cultural context, by exploring how people think through their ideas, and what sorts of constellations of experience inform these complementary practices. Issues of biography, identity, community, and how people within this group thought about their social and cultural positions against the backdrop of migration bring to the forefront the role of biography and community in the management of diabetes, health, and illness. In the following chapter, this biographically situated context to health, culture, race, and diabetes will be discussed further.

References

Ahmad, W. I. U. (1993). *'Race' and health in contemporary Britain*. Buckingham: Open University Press.

Beck, U. (1992). *Risk society – Towards a new modernity*. London: Sage.

Bhopal, R. (1986). The inter-relationship of folk, traditional and Western medicine within an Asian community in Britain. *Social Science and Medicine, 22*(1), 99–105.

Cant, S., & Sharma, U. (1999). *A new medical pluralism?* London: UCL Press.

Cant, S., & Sharma, U. (2003). Alternative health practices and systems. In G. Albrecht, R. Fitzpatrick, & S. Scrimshaw (Eds.), *The handbook of social studies in health and medicine*. London: Sage.

Chacko, E. (2003). Culture and therapy: Complementary strategies for the treatment of type-2 diabetes in an urban setting in Kerala, *India Social Science and Medicine, 56*(5), 1087–1098.

Comelles, J. M., Perdiguero, E., & Martinez-Hernaez, A. (2007). Topographies, folklore and medical anthropology in Spain. In *Medical anthropology: Regional perspectives and shared concerns*. Malden: Blackwell.

Cross, M., & Keith, M. (Eds.). (1992). *Racism, the city and the state*. London: Routledge.

Eade, J. (1997). The power of the experts: The plurality of beliefs and practices concerning health and illness among Bangladeshis in Tower Hamlets, London. In L. Marks & M. Worboys (Eds.), *Migrants, minorities and health: Historical and contemporary studies*. London: Routledge.

Everett, M. (2011). They say it runs in the family: Diabetes and inheritance in Oaxaca, Mexico. *Social Science and Medicine, 72*, 1776–1783.

Farnsworth, N. (1988). Screening plants for new medicines. In E. O. Wilson (Ed.), *Biodiversity*. Washington, DC: National Academy Press. Extract available at: http://www.ciesin.org/docs/002-256c/002-256c.html#fn1. Accessed 21 Oct 2015.

Ferreira, M., & Lang, G. (2006). *Indigenous peoples and diabetes: Community empowerment and wellness*. Durham: Carolina Academic Press.

Gale, N. (2014). The sociology of traditional, complementary and alternative medicine. *Sociology Compass, 8*(6), 805–822. Available at: http://www.pubmedcentral.nih.gov/articlerender.fcgi?artid=4146620&tool=pmcentrez&rendertype=abstract

Giddens, A. (1991). *Modernity and self-identity*. Cambridge: Polity Press.

Helman, C. (1994). *Culture, health and illness* (3rd ed.). Oxford: Butterworth-Heinemann.

Johnston, S. L. (2002). Native American traditional and alternative medicine. *The Annals of the American Academy of Political and Social Science, 583*(1), 195–213.

Kleinman, A. (1988). *The illness narratives: Suffering, healing and the human condition.* New York: Basic Books.

Nettleton, S. (2006). *The sociology of health and illness* (2nd ed.). London: Polity.

Ramakrishna, J., & Weiss, M. G. (1992). Health, illness, and immigration. East Indians in the United States. *The Western Journal of Medicine, 157*(3), 265–270.

Ramji, H. (2006). British Indians 'returning home': An exploration of transnational belongings. *Sociology, 40*(4), 645–662.

Reed, K. (2003). *Worlds of health: Exploring the health choices of British Asian mothers.* London: Praeger.

Saks, M. (1992). *Alternative medicine in Britain.* Oxford: Clarendon Press.

Schutz, A. (1966). Some structures of the life-world. In T. Luckmann (Ed.), *Phenomenology and Sociology.* London: Penguin.

Sharma, U. (1995). *Complementary medicine today, practitioners and patients.* London: Tavistock/Routledge.

Subbulakshmi, G., & Naik, M. (2001). Indigenous foods in the treatment of diabetes mellitus. *Bombay Hospital Journal, 43*, 4.

Wood, D. M., Athwal, S., & Panahloo, A. (2004). The advantages and disadvantages of a 'herbal' medicine in a patient with diabetes mellitus: A case report. *Diabetic Medicine, 21*(6), 625–627.

Worsley, P. (1997). *Knowledges: What different peoples make of the world.* London: Profile Books.

8

Diabetes, Biography, and Community

Introduction

Chapters 6 and 7 have explored two interrelated aspects of the participants' experience of the cultural embedding of type 2 diabetes. The process of being diagnosed, anxieties and fears about diabetes, and help-seeking in biomedical and herbal/traditional forms emerged as integral to a more nuanced view of diabetes. There is also the conceptual and practical juggling that takes place and the locating of this within a cultural context which emerged as themes. This is central to telling the story of people's experiences and demonstrates how people actually respond to the illness, using varieties of experiences, skills, ideas, and methods located and sourced in their lived socialities. Participants, time and again, regardless of the material positions they were observed to be in, are playing out active notions of culture and ethnicity, using all the linguistic, faith, migration experiences, and tools they have in order to negotiate the social and cultural terrain. People are, as they seem to be indicating here, still not 'cultural dopes' (Garfinkel 1984: 68. Certainly, if Avtar Brah's (1996) groundbreaking work on the complexities of South Asian diaspora is to be continuously celebrated, these daily, normalised, routine life–health

© The Editor(s) (if applicable) and The Author(s) 2016
H. Keval, *Health, Ethnicity and Diabetes*,
DOI 10.1057/978-1-137-45703-5_8

activities are part of a deeper embedded fabric of migration and cultural history. As Brah (2007) and others have consistently argued, these bio-graphical identities are not fixed, static, or uni-dimensional. Rather, they are socialities formed in terms of both similarity and difference, which are non-binarised. 'Identity then, is always in process, never an absolutely accomplished fact' (Brah 2007: 139). However, the potential 'unruliness of identity' does not stop social actors from feeling a sense of identity sta-bility, since identity is '…constituted…articulated and expressed through identifications within and across different discourses.' (Brah 2007: 143) I raise these issues at this point in the book because how diabetes—the entire package—is managed by policymakers, service providers, and dia-betics themselves is fundamentally mediated by these processes of iden-tity making.

In this chapter, I further extend this idea with the main focus on how people relate and think about their notions of identity, self, and place, in connection to what they do for their condition. This is not an explicit connection between ethnicity, diabetes, and identity. Rather, it is a more nuanced relationship that emerges when people talk about their condi-tion, how they have managed it, and the kinds of experiences they have had. Many of the respondents arrived in Britain during a time of great social, cultural, and political upheaval—namely, the 1950s to 1970s—often experiencing adversity in varying forms, including racism. Here, the role of biography is important to understanding diabetes contexts. These wider experience 'constellations' (Mason 2002) provide more con-texts about diabetes management against the backdrop of discursively constructed risk. In many ways, identity—the 'who' question which peo-ple ask and answer in different ways—is, if frozen and fixed, a nonsensi-cal notion, because it moulds and changes over time and through space according to certain factors, making it, therefore, contingent and a 'rela-tional' (Bury 2005) idea. As Parekh (2007) has argued, and a point I have made earlier in relation to multicultural citizenship and identity, working within a 'credit-card' notion of identity, where cultural, ethnic, or other 'identities' are seen as moveable and self-contained, results in compart-mentalised and isolated entities. This rendering neglects the nuanced and dynamic realities of lived multiculturality. Ways of being within a given social polity are interlinked, interdependent, and contingent, and this chapter speaks directly to this dynamism in people's biographical management of diabetes.

Given that people experience health and illness, and here, specifically, diabetes in a socially and culturally embedded landscape, the notions of community, place, and biography were important in this study. It is implausible to argue that notions of identity, community, and place, related to life experiences and diabetes management can be separated. Participants demonstrated that ideas of diagnosis, management of diets and exercise, and everyday monitoring of the illness were also bound up with their references to culture, connections to family overseas, references to history in India, as well as the current and immediate connections to local communities. People used both allopathic and traditional herbal remedies in their diabetes management, but also, the combined use of these in terms of general health management. This notion of cultural placement—be it related to one's religion, language, or history—is a prevalent theme in this study, and the use of this 'culturality' as a resource points once more to a more dynamic acting out of social action in people's lived experiences.

The idea of 'biography' has also been used by Carricabburu and Pierret (2002), in their use of Corbin and Strauss's (1987) phrase 'biographical work'. This refers to what an individual needs to do when faced with a chronic illness. In Corbin and Strauss's formulation, 'biographical time', 'conception of self', and 'conception of body' are arranged components which go to make up a biography—it is piecing these together which requires biographical work. Charmaz's (1983) 'loss of self' thesis explored the way in which the self becomes disjointed and fragmented, leaving behind remnants of the once-valued person's self-identity. This, however, could be repaired in what Charmaz (1983) has termed 'reconstituted identities', whereby active participation in the creation of lived experiences was seen as re-forming the once ruptured identity. Similarly, there is a sense in which within this study, participants' many varied diabetes and general health-related activities (here, articulated as 'resistance' to constructions of passivity) can also be regarded as a form of repair to identities. This sense of somehow identifying a disjuncture in one's life—the biography—and then, doing something about it involved two dimensions. One is related to the doing, while the other is related to the narrative account, where certain constructions of the self can be accomplished. Although this work does not concentrate wholly on this narrative account construction, it is relevant because, as Blaxter (2004) argues, narratives allow people to rearrange their experiences, and organise and present their actions, to articulate their place in the world.

The role played by biography within this study is central to the methodological and substantive area in which it sits, since it is only through people's biographies that empirical findings have been asserted. The stories told by people were, in a sense, both a retelling of elements of their lives and a continuous reformation of a notion of social, ethnic, and cultural identity. As Riessman (2001) has argued, narratives are not only personal tellings, but public issues, pointing to social issues that can be addressed. In this sense, and invoking Mills' (1959) argument regarding biography, history, and society, there is a strong notion of the dialectical relationship between agency and structure—that through the reflective appreciation of biographical work, it is possible to address both social structure and the acts within it. Personal experiences of the body in states of illness awareness are juxtaposed with public experiences of, for example, diabetes diagnosis, care, and systems of treatment. Added to this are, of course, the social and cultural milieu within which people act, such as the time period people arrived in this country, experiencing adversity, the issues around finding work, and the coping strategies employed for these problems which permeated their life experiences.

Contextualising the experience of diabetes among the people in this study by looking at biographical features helps to extend the diabetes experience arena (and health and illness sociology, in general) to insights about how a person's own understanding of their 'troubles' can, in turn, be related to social analysis. This, as Riessman (2001) argues, can then be directed to an analysis of larger social complexities or systems. In this study, for example, we can see how a person might go through what might be regarded as routine process of diagnosis, go onto manage their diet and lifestyle, and perhaps, use different remedy systems. Exploring people's own notions of what they do and how they come to think of these actions gives us a clue about the symbolic significance their actions hold. In this study, what I articulate as 'resistance' is a set of actions which constitute culture as dynamic and malleable, and perform complex functions for people to negotiate their landscapes. Their use of various resources then can be gleaned via biographies, and the bonding together of people's histories, identity, and politics through stories (Plummer 1995).

Community and Identity

As shown above, the term 'community' is used to point towards a specific collectivity engaged with physically, practically, and routinely, such as the local community centre. However, a more generalised group notion related to shared religion, language, and caste is also involved. An additional dimension that can be discerned is that of homeland—ideas of identity produced and resultant through the processes of migration. In other words, many people in the sample had strong recollections of their histories and lives before coming to the UK, and their identities were, in part, shaped and influenced by the subsequent experiences they had.

Traversing immediate and extended domains—temporal or spatial—was central to the participants' cultural accomplishment. Interactions with immediate communities as well as wider networks brought about many outcomes, from advice to products, counselling and help. 'Community' here is not to be mistaken for some contrived notion of a Hindu Gujarati collectivity, implying a uniformity and unity within itself, resulting in a version of social closure. Certainly, there are aspects of this that apply, but the term 'community' is used as a much more flexible manifestation of people's social and cultural location. This study was carried out in four locations in the UK, though most of the sample was in two of these locations, which had high concentration of Hindu Gujaratis. Of the remaining two, one has a long history of Hindu Gujarati migration and settlement, while the other has a lesser extent of this demographic. Though it is possible to argue that emphasis in a specific place can reveal the relationship between people, community, and place relations, there is also the risk that this sets up experiences in one or two areas as somehow homogenous and 'authentic', and defends the assumption that by doing so, we are 'tapping' into this entity called 'community'. This study, in part, seeks to break free of contrived notions of 'authentic' community and explore just how wide and elaborate people's own demonstrable ideas of community can be. Malik's (2005) discussion of culture and authenticity is brought to bear here, his critique being that 'authenticity' is a production of Western anthropological quests, whereas for people living within these frameworks, preservation of culture is a lived and required necessity. The importance of a critical stance on 'authenticity' is also emphasised here through the methodology used in the study.

The process of 'cultural validations' clearly sets out the dialectical nature of the researcher–researched relationship as one which can be connected by aspects of ethnic, cultural, linguistic, national, and faith identity. It posits the relationship as precisely that—a relationship, subject to rejections, acceptances, fluid and broken continuities that go towards facilitating the generation of rich data. As well as often being a part of an immediate community, there were wider group memberships within temples and community centres (often the same), which formed a source of identity for people with a strong characterisation of inclusivity, exclusivity, and identity. Often, these communities had multiple identities and subcommunities within them, according to religion, class, caste, and language.

Being Gujarati, Being Diabetic

As discussed earlier, to have diabetes, or '*Sugar nò problem*' (translation: 'the problem of sugar'), was an indicator of a common experience in particular groups. The Gujarati phrase '*Apra ma bho che*', which literally means 'there's a lot of it in ours (our community)', indicates an 'us', which may express a symbolic grouping. The self-reflexive notion that one belongs to, has membership of, and therefore, can—to some extent—utilise services therein, points to a group which is defined by, amongst many other things, the condition of diabetes. This sense of deep historical personal and community-based 'diabetes sense' is not uncommon amongst groups who have been identified as 'high risk'. As Smith-Morris (2006) in her study with Pima Indians in Arizona and Montoya (2011) in his study of Mexican diabetes risk construction found, groups and individuals come to personally and collectively identify their ethnic and cultural ownership of the high-risk package. They do so, however—and as participants here often showed—within a framework of counter-risk narratives that come to exemplify complex articulations of resistance to constructions of passivity.

This commonality or sharing serves as a binding mechanism not only in a social and physical sense—for example, the attendance of weekly over-50s sessions held in local temples—but also conceptually in terms of identity. Ideas of group belonging are rarely limited to a single nationality, country, or similar entity. Participants demonstrated that they had loyalties to a variety of identities—and crucially—they were adhered to and could be called upon when needed. Kanti talked about her undying devotion both to her Hindu faith and to the work of service to others—both being mutually inclusive as ideal states. She explains that as part of her role as a Hindu, she must work in the community in the service of others, helping and assisting people, but she must also uphold the virtues of Hinduism as an organised religion, and utilise her skills that way. While this is an emphasis purely on Hinduism, she also goes on to tell me she moves in 'Muslim' and 'Punjabi' circles (note the mixing of ethno-religious categories), but not as much as the Hindu faith. While this may set up a sense in which there is a preferential treatment of Hindus—given this is the faith she identifies with—this possibility is completely confounded by her demonstrable cultural syncrecy:

> All my neighbours are Muslim, when they come in, I greet them in their custom greeting, and they greet me in my custom greeting. People often ask me 'have you changed religion? Or have you made them into Hindus?' and I say to them, 'yes, they have become Hindus and I have become Muslim'! This is the only way we are able to live, we have to live with one another in this world.

When I asked her how this came to be and why she felt this way, she explained:

> The street we lived in had Hindus, Muslims, different castes, and we all treated each other as a family, always helping, and we tried to make this a daily occurrence...Because you see my father was working under the Europeans, and they used to come to our house to eat, and of course, it was a very mixed environment. We kept our customs in eating and drinking,

and if people eat meat, then we would be seated separately, but it was always with love. We became 'multi'.

It is this 'becoming multi' which draws our attention, since the categorisation of homogenous groups is in favour of simplistic and reified versions of culture and ethnicity. This process, which many of the respondents talk about, here aptly summarised by Kanti as 'becoming multi' indicates that biographies, histories, and experiences outside and within the country, aid and inform how people interact on a daily basis and produce their identities. Within this multifaceted approach is placed the management of health and illness. Examining the fabric of the social context of their illness management points us in the direction of some interesting insights—which direct us to what I articulate here as resistances to constructions of passivity inherent in ideas of the South Asian diabetic risk. The 'multi' process, here expressed as a way of mixing with different cultures, religions, and ethnicities, is not confined just to those participants who explicitly used the term. Rather, this notion of 'multi' is a symbolic link which represents some important processes in the study. The 'becoming multi' can refer to an individual's life course, and perhaps, early experiences through parental exposure to different faith and ethnicity communities, as was the case with Kanti. She employs a network of skills to harness resources, some of these being connections to Hinduism, others more to do with her service work in the community. Her notions of identity are not limited to or restricted by Hinduism, but rather, are part of a wider sense of who she is—the process of 'becoming multi'. The connection to her experience of diabetes, and her health in general, is exemplified here:

No problem! If tomorrow someone says to me I have to live in a small hut, then I'm ready...I go according to circumstances ... anything I can adapt to. My parents trained me to be that way... I go into the books to see why the headache is there, how it should be dealt with.

The 'multi' making appears to be connected to notions of adaptation and survival, so that there are biographical fibres which interconnect at various points in people's lives, and in relation to specific phenomena—

such as illnesses like diabetes. Participants talked of how their life experiences enabled them to deal with the vicissitudes of diabetes as a chronic illness. Certainly, this is not a notion restricted to particular 'ethnic' groups of people. Rather, it is a proccessual element of biography. Life experiences and biographical histories have been revealed to hold many skill sets and enabling structures for the specific and direct everyday management of a condition such as type 2 diabetes, and yet, these skill sets are rarely acknowledged, and more rarely linked to elastic ideas of ethnicity and culture.

As Williams (1993) observed through the framework of 'narrative reconstruction', accounts often demonstrate the pursuit of virtue and moral accomplishments. In this sense, the participants within this study appear to have shown how narratively accounting experience is itself a form of actively engaging the past, present, and possible future by creating forms of one's self—as heard through the medium of storytelling. Through biographies and stories of experience, participants not only demonstrate the possible indications of 'objective' events and experiences, but also indicate proccessual and dynamic account-making in action, through stories of adaptation. This is echoed by Scambler (2002), who observes that narratives are cognitive schemes, constructed in time and space, which serve a function of maintaining a coherent whole. Here, the coherency required is made more critical because of the way in which diabetes is embedded within wider arenas of social experience. In the case of Deena, her early experiences in the UK led her to much voluntary work, helping in the South Asian community, cooking, organising, and helping in many other ways, and as she explains, this was very much a multicultural environment:

> Years ago, I used to help this centre, even in heavy snow, we used to walk, make food, and help. We never took any money for any of this, it was for the community. Then finally, a grant was available, and it grew. At first, it was just us Gujaratis, then it grew to Muslims, Punjabis, and it became mixed. They then moved to another area…Well, it was too far me to travel to.

In her account, Deena is linking collective identity and group cohesion in the face of migration to a new country, with the ability and capacity of the embodied 'self'—which has now undergone changes due to illness and age. These experiences are not confined to historical notions of the past, nor limited to memories of a particular geographical place, such as India or Africa, but are very much a lived contemporary concept. The account reflects a process, dynamic with social and biographical activity, and current utilisation of knowledge rather than a snapshot of history. The processes and phenomena discussed in Chaps. 6 and 7, and as we can see here, the integrated notions of pre- and post-migration experiences as providing a 'support base' are bound together. The sense in which these elements cannot be separated and treated as reified objects supports the idea that within collectivities and individual lives, illness and health management is taking a dynamic form through the utilisation of resources available to people. These resources, rather than being external to people, are woven into their biographies and are called upon to negotiate personal and social experiences. This demonstration of a multicultural layering of social networks is not confined to either the South Asian group or subgroups. As Harish tells me, he has a curiosity and a 'need to know', which is part of his overall make-up, but which also informs his diabetes management:

> I go everywhere! I go to the church assembly, Gurdwara, temple…Just out of interest…just to know about other people…at the church assembly and Gurdwara, I talk with them and, many times, I can clear up their misunderstanding about Hinduism.

Certainly, as Harish and others talked and narrated their many different daily or intermittent engagement with various religious contexts, what emerges in the manner of these encounters is the relative ease with which the multiplicity of interconnected relations facilitates people's health and social life management. Turner's (2015) characterisation of societies that have modified and adapted to larger overarching changes to globalisation of culture and capital is useful here. The change from 'sticky' societies, where engagement, access, and exit from membership involves high investment and high cost, to societies that are more 'elastic', where this engagement has lesser cost to the individual, may not strictly apply here, but there are elements of organised, ritual practice, interactions requiring acknowledgement of spiritual and bureaucratic hierarchies that people are cognisant of. However, the deeply personal, and personalised, nature of their religious and spiritual beliefs allows them to perform a wide variety of elasticities, in accordance with the needs of specific situations and contexts.

Adversity and Coping

Repeating Bhopal's (2006) assertion in the opening chapter that the key to understanding the health of minority populations is in understanding migration, I extend this call and argue for what medical anthropologists such as Montoya (2011), Ferreira and Lang (2006), Scheper-Hughes (2006), and others have long called for. That is a multifaceted, biographical, and socio-cultural picture of illness sufferers, which can adequately, and in a nuanced way, trace the myriad microprocesses and impacts of wider structural forces on individual and group lives. In this book, I have tried to attend to this by exploring the overarching discourses which construct 'risky' identities and, in parallel, look towards the dynamic socially and culturally negotiated nature of health and illness management. Situating illness experience within the biographical details of people's lives is important to understand how they might think of diabetes, and negotiate the illness. The phrase 'becoming multi' denotes the notion of a sense of multicultural adaptation, which existed long before the discourses of race, ethnicity, and difference became popular in post-war Britain. This adaptation, as the participants show, indicates that there is a coping style and management method that is used by people to deal with a variety of situations arising in their lives, including diabetes. This connection is perhaps plausible as a way of linking their experiences of racism and hardship, with the adversity experienced by their neighbours during the war years. The connection is further extended by explaining that while things were certainly difficult in the early days, it was people of Harish's generation who were helpful:

It would be one house, and 7–10 people living in there at once. You got to know people, where they were from, who they were. In 1958–60 you couldn't even find a place to live here, a house. No shop, no house, even if you had money, they wouldn't sell you a house, couldn't get a mortgage, we'd burn coals in the house and be bathing in the public baths!

As with many other studies that examine the experience of chronic illness in people's lives (e.g. Anderson and Bury 1988; Bury 2001; Charmaz 2000), this study looks at the location of a particular chronic illness in the everyday lives of people who live with it. A variety of contextual issues emerged in the interviews. For example, when I asked Deena about how long she and her family had been in the country, she talked about how she had been widowed quite early in the move to the UK, and then, about her and her family's experiences of violent racism. She talked about how they had to move within the same city, to different areas, because of racism, and other difficult living conditions:

> After my son had been attacked, we moved…I didn't feel safe there anymore. There were all sorts of people hanging around, and I was alone with my young son…we moved, and unfortunately, there were a lot of ruffians and yobs in the area. When I was working part-time, I was coming home from work, and they would shout 'paki', and bullied my son at college as well. Then, we sold the house, and moved here. Here, we're happy, and have peace.

Deena's interview was often characterised by her sense of adaptation and survival, borne out of her experiences in India, but also, the adverse migration settlement experiences in the UK. This was placed in a framework of living, which acknowledged the constraints she was under as a migrant in a new country, and the active cultural negotiations that would be required in her dealings with people from different communities and faith. Through this framework, she could manage her diabetes using a variety of mechanisms, as did many of the participants in different ways. Not only do chronic illness sufferers have to live with the physical and psychosocial impact of the illness on their lives, but in the case of 'minority' populations, there is the added obstacle of racism and risk of violence in their everyday lives (e.g. Nazroo 1997; IRR 2015; Craig et al. 2012).

As emphasised within this study, the role of 'structures of relevance' (Schutz 1962) gives an indication that biographical contexts are employed in making sense of the world, and used in ways which allow the management of conditions like diabetes in a taken-for-granted fashion. Coping with an illness then may well be part of the overall panoply of life events which people need to negotiate and deal with, especially when there are a range of difficulties relating to race and racism to manage. Some of the people in the sample were able to relate their experiences of adversity to their management of their diabetes, health, and illness in general while others did not specifically emphasise this coping strategy. For people like Sunita (aged 70), adversity was indeed a part of everyday life, and being a widow, living alone and in an area where she shared neither language nor culture with the residents, diabetes was another situation to deal with. However, as shown in earlier chapters, this has a bearing on our current discussion of biography and identity. Despite the obstacles, Sunita demonstrated that embedded in her everyday living are mechanisms for managing adversity, such as visiting the local community centre. This is something she is unsure of, but feels is beneficial, visiting the local 'Indian' shopping area where she can meet with people and talk, and as shown later, her religious faith framework. Here, Reed's 'layers of community' (2003: 165) is a useful way to look at the identity and structure management system for participants as they move along, within and outside of axes of different types of belonging, simultaneously informed by the parallel management of health and illness. Within these layers of resources, which are utilised in various ways at various times, diabetes is one of a range of problems that need to be addressed:

> I never used to go much but people said to me I should go, meet people, learn things. These days, I do go…There are people there, you can meet them, see their faces, it makes your heart happier, and you can have a nice time, talking to people… There are no Indians here. But having been here 25 years, I'm used to it. Sometimes, I go, sit there, and meet people… For the last 8–10 years, I've not taken sugar in my tea, no other sweet stuff; you have to take care of yourself. People at the hospital often tell me that I look after myself, and that I have courage. Sometimes, it does get bad, but that's the way it is with diabetes.

I always go outside. Afternoons, I'm always out, I do my prayers, then cook whatever I need to and then leave the house for a while…I still go… whatever one can do for one self, one must, just maintain courage.

Embedded within Sunita's account are numerous themes, connecting her methods of dealing with her social landscapes, from getting exercise, socialising, maintaining her diet, to talking about the need to be as self-sufficient as possible, given the generational and lifestyle differences between family members. This, of course, strikes many resonant chords with the documented experiences of migrants to Britain in the early post-war years (Visram 2002; Ballard 1994). It also invites a more multifaceted approach to exploring health and illness, and the intersections with ethnicity and culture. In Part 1, I outlined the various limitations of many prevailing approaches to this area, some of which took culture and ethnicity to be discrete, fixed snapshots in people's lives, and that, once captured as an identity characteristic within so-called 'race-health' research, would be applied in a reified fashion. In Sunita's and other participants' talk, what we can see is the demonstrative complexity of everyday negotiations in health and illness.

Religion, 'Higher Power' and Health

As participants were Gujarati people mostly of the Hindu faith, most were located and approached through local temples and community centres and through a popular cultural and religious event. This runs the risk of making a set of assumptions: that all the people in the sample are followers of the same faith; that it was not necessary to look beyond these locations, employing a 'one-size-fits-all' stereotype; and that religion would not be a discussion point in the interview since it was a taken-for-granted entity. Religion here is not used in a narrow, categorical sense, but as an example of cultural context. The physical and social borders created and used by people was an interesting element here. Whilst aware of the importance of place and identity relations, there was also an awareness of artificial notions of 'community' and place limited to one temple where people might gather, and become the researcher's focus. Religion was indeed not raised by me in any of the interviews, except one, but was mostly raised by the participants themselves, as shown below.

Much research has been carried out in the field of spirituality and health (Labun and Emblen 2007) and the relationship between them. At one research site, the duality of the specific location was interesting, since there was no explicit revealing of 'religious-ness', and therefore, there appeared to be a 'secular clause' available to attendees of the centre. For those requiring explicit religious devotion, there was a fully functioning temple, where people could go and worship. Here, some of the participants talked about how much help and support they gained from their religion:

> I was never worried. Once, I had 5 complications in the stomach, a serious operation, and I was unconscious for 9 days. At that time, I saw a big light, I have a memory of the light, and even today, when I remember, it makes me happy. God is with me, my faith is strong. Whenever I have a question or dilemma, all I do is pray overnight, and the next day, I usually have an answer. (Kanti)
>
> I've just let God take care of my illness. Diabetes, arthritis, I have it all. Still, I'm ok. God keeps me well. Without the grace of God, nothing can happen, he controls everything, so I just put faith in him, and he takes care of me, and gives me courage. I get courage from God, and I don't feel alone. I've been here 25 years, and there have been burglaries everywhere around here, except here (my home). (Sunita, 70)
>
> I've always been quite spiritual, I've always believed, and I believe in certain things and that's where my strength comes from. I don't pray every day, but I'll say a little something. We don't go to temples, we have one at home. To me, God is everywhere; you don't have to go to a specific place. (Rina)

The role of religious belief is not an all-encompassing ontology which operates exclusively, but rather, in the context of participant's lives, works with and between other support structures. For Kanti, while describing unshakeable faith, the life lived well and virtuously is one where the individual utilises her surroundings for the purpose of doing good—this automatically includes self-preservation, survival through adverse circumstances, and proper management of illnesses. As she stated, *'You have to be your own doctor and treat your body in a way which pleases you.'*

In a way similar to the use of herbal remedies and cultural knowledge, her religion provided a method of finding solace and comfort whilst at the same time it also functioned as a cultural reproduction and maintenance tool, used to facilitate a religious, but also a 'healthy' and 'virtuous' (Blaxter 2004) identity. However, leaving diabetes to God is not an indication of fatalism or passivity. On the contrary, it acts more like Schutz's (1970) zones of relevance—as a support mechanism, which increases the likelihood of actively negotiating health and illness, through whatever means is possible. The existing community centres which provide meeting points, lunch, health education talks, and a social focus for the people here are evidence that organised religious frameworks are a useful tool for collective mobilisation. The use of religious and faith systems, spiritual frameworks, organised or otherwise, is widely known to be used to aid recovery from a range of health problems. Where the intersection with ethnicity and culture is apparent, studies have shown that these spiritual frameworks, as they interact with identity, have been crucial (Morjaria-Keval and Keval 2015). Although all of these participants talked of faith and religion as powerful support mechanisms, they also all demonstrated that their religious ideas were embedded within a wider social fabric. Contrary to some research carried out in South Asian communities—which depicts people as passive and fatalistic recipients of religious belief (Naeem 2003) —here, people are reflexive co-producers of social action. Religion is part of their overall framework for dealing with diabetes. Using religion as one of many resources led to a multifaceted interactional model of their daily lives, rather than a unitary model. The invoking and implementation of religious/faith belief systems did not appear here as a rigid or reductive limitation on people's agency and therefore ability to traverse the complexities of health and illness. Rather, as an embodied social and cultural process, as Turner (2014) highlights in his review of sociological approaches to religion, it transcends the limited notions, and perhaps, conventional models of religion as merely a collection of values and beliefs, towards an inherently embodied sense of ritual, materiality, and a knowledge and respect for place (Rey 2007).

Conclusion

Within participants' socialities, there is a complex set of relations between the local and global, the immediate and extended environment, and the past and present. These dialectics also extend to notions of how people located themselves in terms of self-identity. Although all participants regarded themselves as Gujarati, they all utilised a weaving of multiple identities for social accomplishment, but also for the purposes of diabetes management. The multivocality with which participants expressed their notions of identity within their social and cultural experiences was also extended beyond both physical and conceptual borders. Through talking about managing diabetes and community interactions, they were able to negotiate a range of experiences using the cultural and ethnic resources they had available—which included biographical and life experiences. Participants found ways in which notions of passivity are bypassed, and their cultural and ethnic identity frameworks were employed to deal with their illness as a lived and embodied occurrence. The kinds of remedies, medicines, and balancing of nutrition needs are also presented as complex webs of interaction, whereby people reflect upon the impacts of nutrition and activity on their diabetes, but do so within the structures of their own life histories, narratives, and experiences. Notions of identity and place as lived entities were weaved into the diabetes experience and situated the accounts in relation to other structures, which are used to buffer the diabetes experience. Connected to these were other structures, such as religion and faith, experiences of racism, and links to people in the community. If we can identify a series of discursive constructions of South Asian risk in the diabetes arena, what people actually do, as shown here, often runs counter to this narrative. People's social and cultural activities within the management of diabetes can be identified as forms of 'resistance' to the constructions of passivity and cultural pathology as described above. These resistances are demonstrably manifested as active negotiations of health and illness, and more accurately, cultural negotiations. Within their lived social contexts, participants were using the resources in their life histories, experiences of adversity in migration, and their experiences in their 'origin' countries, as well as their current and immediate connections to communities around them, as enabling and empowering structures.

In the following chapter, I return to and address some of the core components of the discursive racialised constructions of South Asian diabetes—namely, the racial-genetic diabetes risks as conceptualised in the discourse. In a sense, this genetic understanding, following on from the previous three chapters, frames the nature of the complexity in this subject. The accounts and practices of the people as shown in their talk and actions are inherently socially and culturally malleable, expressive of the movement and fluidity within all social lives. 'Ethno-racial' diabetes understandings, as they are interwoven with a reimagining of the biological through 'new genetics', alert us to the way in which essentialist and reductionist knowledge making processes re-emerge in a cyclical fashion. I turn to these issues now, in Chap. 9.

References

Anderson, R., & Bury, M. (1988). *Living with chronic illness: The experience of patients and their families*. London: Unwin Hyman.

Ballard, R. (1994). *Desh Pardesh: The South Asian presence in Britain*. London: Hurst.

Bhopal, R. (2006). Race and ethnicity: Responsible use from epidemiological and public health perspectives. J Law Med Ethics. Fall, *34*(3), 500–7, 479.

Blaxter, M. (2004). Life narratives, identity and health. In D. Kelleher & G. Leavy (Eds.), *Identity and health*. London: Routledge.

Brah, A. (1996). *Cartographies of Diaspora: Contesting identities*. London: Routledge.

Brah, A. (2007). Non-binarised identities of similarity and difference. In M. Wetherall, M. Lafleche, & R. Berkeley (Eds.), *Identity, ethnic diversity and community cohesion*. London: Sage

Bury, M. (2001). Illness narratives: Fact or fiction? *Sociology of Health & Illness, 23*(3), 263–285.

Bury, M. (2005). *Health – A short introduction*. Cambridge: Polity Press.

Carricabburu, D., & Pierret, J. (2002). From biographical disruption to biographical reinforcement: The case of HIV positive men. In S. Nettleton & U. Gustavson (Eds.), *The sociology of health and illness reader*. Cambridge: Polity Press.

Charmaz, K. (1983). Loss of self: A fundamental form of suffering in the chronically ill. *Sociology of Health and Illness, 5*, 168–195.

Charmaz, K. (2000). Experiencing chronic illness. In G. Albrecht, R. Fitzpatrick, & S. Scrimshaw (Eds.), *The handbook of social studies in health and medicine.* London: Sage.

Corbin, J., & Strauss, A. L. (1987). Accompaniments of chronic illness: Changes in body, self, biography and biographical time. *Research in the Sociology of Health Care, 6*, 249–281.

Craig, G., Atkin, K., Chatoo, S., & Flynn, R. (Eds.). (2012). *Understanding 'race' and ethnicity: Theory, history, policy, practice.* Bristol: Policy Press.

Ferreira, M., & Lang, G. (2006). *Indigenous peoples and diabetes: Community empowerment and wellness.* Durham: Carolina Academic Press.

Garfinkel, H. (1984). *Studies in ethnomethodology.* Cambridge: Polity Press.

Institute of Race Relations. (2015). http://www.irr.org.uk/. Accessed 21 Oct 2015.

Labun, E., & Emblen, J. D. (2007). Spirituality and health in Punjabi Sikh. *Journal of Holistic Nursing: Official Journal of the American Holistic Nurses' Association, 25*(3), 141–148; discussion 149–150. Available at: http://www.ncbi.nlm.nih.gov/pubmed/17724380. Accessed 26 Nov 2014.

Malik, K. (2005). Making a difference: Culture, race and social policy. *Patterns of Prejudice, 39*(4), 361–378.

Mason, J. (2002). *Qualitative interviewing.* London: Sage.

Mills, C. W. (1959). *The sociological imagination.* New York: Oxford University Press.

Montoya, M. J. (2011). *Making the Mexican diabetic: Race, science, and the genetics of inequality.* London: University of California Press.

Morjaria-Keval, A., & Keval, H. (2015). Reconstructing Sikh spirituality in recovery from alcohol addiction. *Religions, 6*(1), 122–138.

Naeem, A. G. (2003). The role of culture and religion in the management of diabetes: A study of Kashmiri men in Leeds. *The Journal for the Royal Society for the Promotion of Health, 123*(2), 110–116.

Nazroo, J. (1997). *The health of Britain's ethnic minorities: Findings from a national survey.* London: Policy Studies Institute.

Parekh, B. (2007). Reasoned identities: A committed relationship. In M. Wetherall, M. LaFleche, & R. Berkeley (Eds.), *Identity, ethnic diversity and community cohesion.* London: Sage.

Plummer, K. (1995). *Telling sexual stories: Power, change, and social worlds.* London: Routledge.

Reed, K. (2003). *Worlds of health: Exploring the health choices of British Asian mothers.* London: Praeger.

Rey, T. (2007). *Bourdieu on religion: Imposing faith and legitimacy.* London: Equinox.

Riessman, C. K. (2001). Personal troubles as social issues: Narrative of infertility in context. In I. Shaw & N. Gould (Eds.), *Qualitative researching in social work.* London: Sage.

Scambler, G. (2002). *Health and social change.* Buckingham: Open University Press.

Scheper-Hughes, N. (2006). Diabetes and genocide-beyond the thrifty gene. In M. Ferreira & G. Lang (Eds.), *Indigenous peoples and diabetes: Community empowerment and wellness.* Durham: Carolina Academic Press.

Schutz, A. (1970). *Reflections on the problem of relevance.* New Haven: Yale University Press.

Smith- Morris, C. (2006). *Diabetes among the Pima: Stories of survival.* Tucson: University of Arizona Press.

Turner, B. S. (2014). *Religion and contemporary sociological theories. Current Sociology,* 62(6), 771–778.

Visram, R. (2002). *Asians in Britain: 400 years of history.* London: Pluto.

Williams, G. (1993). Chronic illness and the pursuit of virtue in everyday life. In A. Radley (Ed.), *World of illness: Biographical and cultural perspectives on health and disease.* London: Routledge.

9

'Race-ing' Back to the Bio-genetic Future?

The inclination towards the end of the book is to engage with a conventional intellectual academic process which presents this work in a linear fashion, such that having provided a series of discursive constructional backdrops, the book then proceeds to unpack and deconstruct those formations. The aim was to show that constructions of 'risk' within South Asian populations as they are configured in cultural, lifestyle, and genetic science are performing specific and wide-ranging functions. These functions serve to mask the often vaguely conceptualised and operationalised notions of 'culture', 'ethnicity', 'race', and even manage to confuse geopolitical categories with ethno-religious and linguistic ones. On the basis of this and other themes I have discussed, there was a need to deconstruct these formulations because they have far-reaching consequences for the populations in question. Part of this narrative 'set-up' for the book was to address briefly, in early chapters, the scientific formulations of genetic predisposition in the so-labelled racial category, 'South Asian'. The linear trajectory of conventional narrative requires that I leave the material where I discussed it, and move to closure by progressing to a conclusion. I would like to resist this temptation, and re-alert readers to the view that the 'genetic race chapter' in public health, diabetes research,

© The Editor(s) (if applicable) and The Author(s) 2016
H. Keval, *Health, Ethnicity and Diabetes*,
DOI 10.1057/978-1-137-45703-5_9

and academic quarters is hardly closed, and re-emerges as newly formulated, albeit bringing with it older tropes of racial inequality. Within this chapter, I am opening the door onto a vista of future possibilities in which race and raciological meaning-making make their presence felt. The great 'treacherous bind', which Rhadakrishnan (1996) identified in both utilising race categories to explore the multiple ways in which they work, whilst simultaneously informing us that we are, indeed, complicit in the very process we are attempting to define and condemn, is appropriate here. I revisit the area of race-genetics diabetes arguments here precisely because the way 'race-thinking' re-emerges in different forms at different times within discursive formations is powerful and insidious in its shape-shifting mechanisms.

In Chap. 4 I provided a context for genetic arguments in South Asian diabetes discourse in order to situate and frame this component of the discourse within the schema of interrelated risk constructions. This broad range of knowledge-making formations necessarily works in interconnected ways, and as with all statements or indications within a 'discursive formation' (Foucault 1972: 38) they rely on each other and support a common purpose, which is the production of knowledge, and the use of practice to further this knowledge-making (Hall and Gieben 1992). The temptation I refer to above—to regard racial-genetics as a separate component of the overall picture—is to be resisted because the multiple weavings of the racialised fabric of society and health cannot possibly be rendered analytically clear in such a linear fashion. It is precisely because of its nature as complex and problematic, 'fictive', 'relational', and 'fluid' (Bloch et al. 2013) that it re-emerges from the psychosocial comfort of 'cultural' explanations of health inequalities and disparities. It manifests within genetic arguments as reasonable, scientifically legitimate, and therefore, outside the realms of critique. Having never really disappeared, race presents itself through various forms of discursive practice and 'categorising tendencies' (Gunaratnam 2003: 30) via a 'cultural recoding' (Bloch et al. 2013), as a 'newly' formed, 'floating signifier' (Hall 1996). It is adorned with the paraphernalia of high-tech, biogenetic science, whilst underneath, carefully concealing older, troubling cultural-raciological meanings.

To elaborate this process here, I emphasise and provide some detail of the *fluid*, intellectual process in which race-genetic arguments in South Asian diabetes discourse have a paradoxically *reifying* nature. I willingly and inconclusively conclude my book with a series of issues and emergent urgencies regarding the development of this racio-genetic argument in South Asian diabetes discourse, firm in the knowledge that the danger and risks of not being vigilant to this form of re-essentialising are serious and potentially wide-ranging.

The core concerns of this book are made salient through the revisiting of the race–genetics argument at this point, and first, illustrate its relevance for the analysis of racialised discursive constructions of risk, and second, show that whilst development in gene-science technology are constantly (as one might expect) moving forward, the genetic predisposition argument is far from new. The genetic argument, as I show in Chap. 4, was a feature of the early stages of diabetes and health analysis, and cyclically continues to be reinvested into institutional scientific discourse, through more subtle variations on the theme, such as gene–environment, or gene–culture interactions. 'Race-ing' towards this supposed safer, ontological, and epistemological comfort of gene–environment or genetic predisposition theories only renders the arena with a murkier, bio-raciological hue. Elsewhere (Keval 2015), I have developed in some detail these arguments, and here, I summarise and discuss pertinent issues. We can resituate the cultural and lifestyle ethno-diabetes risk package I refer to in this book, and view the way in which subjects are responsible, and therefore, partly culpable in their choices of 'cultural' health behaviour and lifestyles. However, the often vaguely and poorly conceptualised notions of ethnicity, culture, and intersectional factors means that this 'fact-file' (Gunaratnam 2003) approach to identity and health offers very few *certainties* for health policy, intervention, and academia. As active owners of 'risky cultures', these same subjects can, however, be viewed as passive owners of 'risky genes' through a new era of biogenetic science. By mobilising this newfound enthusiasm for race-genetics in the name of health, a still as yet precarious scientific truth claim has gained profound traction. This is something I have called the dialectic of 'certain-uncertainty' knowledges.

The elaboration or 'evolution of medical uncertainty' (Fox 1980) has a long history and is now well-established as a general analytical principle within medical sociology internationally. For Fox, the honest and critical reflection of being uncertain about the limits of medical science, knowledge, training, and expertise were built into the process of training as a doctor (Fox 1957), and she developed many of the classic medical sociological themes of the time. For writers who explore this area, there is a necessary relationship between certainty and uncertainty, because acknowledging this reality facilitates mechanisms to cope—whether this is to mobilise professional integrity or to secure a better client–professional relationship (1980). Indeed, in this type of analysis, one can observe the ways in which healthcare professionals are constantly embedded in the processes of the human condition—in a phrase, the core of meaning-making within life, as illness, death, physical and mental deterioration call into question some of the fundamental aspects of ontological insecurity. Although Fox's early writing and subsequent work are wide-ranging and have focused on clinical work, it does help us cut to a core issue in the subject of this book. The analytical problem of uncertainty in biomedicine, here extended to the various racial-genetic lenses, can be concerned with the relationship between what is knowable—and therefore currently certain—and what is unknowable—and therefore uncertain. I do not separate these as distinct categories, but rather, question the very way in which what can be known, and what cannot be known, are re-envisaged and conceptualised in order to generate what I have called certain-certainties. The classification of South Asian genetic diabetes risk is part of this reconceptualisation of 'knowability'. Whilst the built-in coping with of the 'uncertainty-about-uncertainty' (Fox 1980: 44) reflects the ambivalent, even reflective, nature of the intellectual and professional practice of medicine (other established critiques notwithstanding, e.g. Illich 1976, Navarro 1978), in our case, there is a difference. The demonstrative performativity of racial-genetic explanations are certain about their certainties—despite the precarious conceptualisations on which this knowledge sits.

As I mention earlier in Chap. 4, there has yet to be a conclusive, empirical, evidence base to a definitive genetic marker for diabetes. What is, therefore, fascinating is that given the identical nature of 99.9 % of the human genome (Ossorio and Duster 2005; Montoya 2011), there is a profoundly robust investment (both financial and ideological) in the intellectual and discursive industry surrounding race-genetic research into diabetes. This 0.01 % difference in genetic material is a miniscule entity for geneticists to generate and derive wide-ranging statements regarding genetic predisposition amongst populations defined by categories sourced in geopolitical, social, cultural, and economic categorisations. The underlying proposition to the genetic work is still Neel's 'thrifty genotype' (1962) argument, revisited and revised by the author himself. What I would like to do here is address some of the themes I mentioned in Chap. 4, namely, the certainty–uncertainty tension in race-genetic diabetes science, and racialised discursive constructions of risk therein, because of the differential impact on groups.

It is the curious ambivalence of the type of knowledge demonstrated by, for example, Gholap et al. (2011), as mentioned earlier, that is remarkable in its power to seduce using constructed racial certainties. This is despite a range of work reviewing scientific evidence (Hartley 2014) for the efficacy of genetic risk profiling in screening programmes indicating no additional payoffs in health indicators. It is the *possibility* alone of a genetic certainty which drives much of this discursivity in its truth claims, the symbolic and practical significance of which are part of the ethno-diabetes package. This possibility is mobilised in a starkly 'certain' manner, demonstrating a performance of absolute security in the knowledge base. This type of 'genetic Black-boxing of race' (Morning 2014: 1681) is readily available in genetic science discourse, and presumes an unquestioning validity and truth in its presentation and operation, especially when allied to the disciplines working in 'public health' and 'ethnic inequalities'. Although Bhopal's (2013) 'four stage' model explaining higher risk of diabetes amongst South Asians appears ostensibly to be a considered gene–environment interaction model (Seabrook and Avison 2010), there are issues which need addressing. The linear trajectory of the 4-stage model, which starts with the 'small…fatty baby' (2013: 36), and progressively moves through a series of stages ending in the deterioration of beta cells, also includes *lifestyle choices* such as 'low physical activity' (2013: 36). The gene–environment interaction appears to be a combination of absolute genetic weakness (gene), combined with a relative social and cultural deficit (environment), resulting in higher risks and patterns of incidence and prevalence. While Bhopal (2013) calls for a multifactorial approach comprising environmental, social, and cultural mechanisms, the emergent salience appears in the form of the gene. I draw attention to this not to contest the viability of various complexities of genetic science, or indeed, any interventions intended to improve access to healthcare services or information. Rather, I highlight the ways in which social practices facilitate meaning construction and related notions of validity. As the social, scientific, and philosophical analysis of medicine bears out, ideals of scientific objectivity and value-freedom characterising the biomedical hegemony parallel similar patterns of legitimacy claims in genetic science. This has a specific set of consequences for racialised health status. In addition, the innocuous and apparently compromise-laden gene–environment framework is, as Happe (2013) has elaborated, fundamentally flawed. By normalising those structural practices that result in inequalities, the concept of 'susceptibility' is situated within the discourse, thereby creating the possibility of 'small subsets of "truly" at-risk individuals' whose only real, effective course of acceptable and legitimate action in terms of help-seeking is 'actionable knowledge confined to practices of the body in the private sphere… (these) practices include therapies to counteract susceptibility' (Happe 2013: 180). Whilst Happe refers to some of the insidious and damaging effects of industrial capitalism and pollution, it is not difficult to extend her argument to the ways in which the ethno-racial South Asian diabetes risk is caught within the benevolent sounding complications of so-called gene–environment interactions.

Whilst acknowledging that scientific knowledge bases are themselves often rarely uni-dimensional, reflectively accommodating tensioned relationships between hegemonic normalisations and 'spaces of resistance and counter hegemony' (Keval 2015: 8), there is an enduring requirement for vigilance. Where race, culture, ethnicity, power, and health intersect, these discursively identified spaces can be reduced and limited in their ability to offer opportunities for resistance. It is difficult, after all, to argue with 'genetic truths', especially when represented in systems of scientific, healthcare provision and official government discourse. There are, therefore, some interesting and potentially contradictory components of the 'ethno-racial' diabetes risk in South Asians, as exemplified in Bhopal's work. Although steadfastly critical of approaches which ignore the potential harm in narrow biological-focused explanations, these models often redirect the firmly established social, cultural, and economic arguments towards genetic models of causality. The use of evolutionary models 'out of step with modern lifestyle' (2013: 37), 'cultural' peculiarities in South Asian preferences, and emphases on 'the enjoyment of good tasty food … at the heart of family life, and hospitality towards family and friends' (ibid.) is highly problematic. It highlights one of the core aims of this book, specifically to warn against the continued cultural patholigisation of South Asian cultures, and here, its expedient combination with genetic reification. Cultural practices, frameworks for negotiating the complexities of everyday social life are embedded inside the practices of all social beings and groups—as is the social, cultural, and economically (Schubert et al. 2012) mediated nature of food consumption and engagement therein. It is not a statically categorised 'racial' or 'ethnic' 'disposition' to be used to describe, or indeed, analyse specific groups with the intention of demarcating causal fault lines for complex health disorders.

The cultural/lifestyle arguments I discuss in earlier chapters is combined with genetic scientific discourse, resulting in particular constructions of a 'risk package' mobilising cultural pathology as well as culpable genetic material. With culture and lifestyle, the subjects can make choices (and we remain cognisant of the mediated and contingent nature of 'choice') through various changes and modifications to health choices, and/or 'cultural' frameworks. There is, therefore, potentially directed culpability, which remains within the group, whilst genetic predispositions result in what Montoya (2011) calls the ethno-racial geneticisation of diabetes. Whilst foregoing culpability, genetic arguments with inherent scientific infallibility suggest essentialist reductionism, down to the molecular level. This facilitates notions of certainty and ontological security, allowing little room for the lived dynamics of everyday life that we associate with culture. Culture, therefore, becomes the troublesome and unstable counterpart to the more certainty-ridden and better manageable racial gene.

One question that might be raised here is perhaps connected to the inevitability of technical progress in gene–environment or genetic science, and that, surely conceptualisations of social life necessarily need to acknowledge and accommodate the genetic and genomic (Novas and Rose 2000a, b). Certainly, discussions about the genetic possibilities in South Asian diabetes risk could feasibly be entertained under a more general umbrella of societal change, something Novas and Rose (ibid) call 'somatic individuality'. Within this gaze, social and cultural life moves from the outwardly focused individual and group-focused experiences, to the more ultra-interior-based focus of molecular visions. New forms of biomedical knowledge, language, and ways to describe people, rather than objectifying and reducing agency, actually give birth to agency and effect empowerment. Just as physical, somatic conditions result in the bearer being involved in the clinical encounter as a co-producer of the knowledge and decision-making process, in the lay–professional relationship, there are, supposedly, parallels within these new genetic forms of understanding social life. Thus, there are potentially various ways in which people can have some control and power in the negotiated order of the medical situation, and thereby, can mitigate any uncertainties involved through partnerships with genetic science. As a hypothetical ideal, this has some normative merit, but in the case of race, ethnicity, and diabetes, there are many problems, and they are related to my overall concerns in this chapter of the relationship between race, power, and health.

A 'Genetic optimism' (Conrad and Gabe 1999) performs a form of ideological function here, such that we need to interrogate this agency-empowering new genetic citizenship. What evidence is there that when we intersect experiences of health and illness with race, ethnicity, culture, class, and power, the groups that have traditionally been at the subjugated polarity of the continuum actually are enabled to take more control in the categorisations, diagnostics, prognosis, and treatments for their conditions? And where the issue is deemed part of the genetic 'ethno-racial' South Asian diabetes package, what possible preventative components might be considered? Having control over one's health, as social science has firmly established, involves multiple layers of social, economic, and cultural positioning. Certainly, there are many unanswered questions about the possible impact of racialised geneticisation of South Asian people with diabetes, when we consider the interactive points in GP surgeries, hospitals, clinics, and other healthcare contexts. It is in these contexts that race, knowledge, and power play out in the social and cultural drama of health identities. Experts and care providers will come to understand and disseminate what they believe to be irrefutable genetic truths about racial categories of people. Subjects at the receiving end of this information may not necessarily be in positions to contest and refute such fallibility, and may not be in positions where they can relate to these new forms of social genetic 'being', as described by some authors. How might people even contemplate refuting genetic racial categorisation, especially if language, education, and social class are major differentials? The fluidity and situational nature of all identities notwithstanding, there are enduring material relations that mediate power and knowledge production, and the resultant 'race making' articulations (Knowles 2007). Genetic race-making could indeed potentially exacerbate problems within the negotiations of diabetes for minority groups by increasing what Aspinall (2013) identifies as the stigmatising and discriminatory possibilities of genetic labelling. Although prominent authors in the field of genetics and society point out, for example, that 'variation is the norm' (Rose 2009: 11), emphasising the nuanced view that genomic work is complex and multifactorial, nevertheless, the 'democratization of genetic knowledge' (Keval 2015: 11) is not necessarily open to all groups in society. As the contemporary quest for certainty and stability in knowledge requires technology as a principle progress driver, it is both genetic racialised hegemony that I warn against and the associated differential impacts with few opportunities for contestation that become a concern.

Stating that contemporary forms of 'biological citizenship' (Rose and Novas 2007) allow, and indeed, drive forward networks of newly emergent, informed, and empowered identities, involving family, clinicians, and other mediators of biomedical and genetic knowledge does not appear to acknowledge the many enduring and multiple forms of disenfranchisement that can result from racialisation. To be placed under an 'ethno-racial' gaze focusing on one's South Asian diabetes risk vulnerability is a racial discursive formation that inherently situates people in this grouping as bearers of a particularly troublesome package of health identities. The tensioned relationship between possibly refutable cultural pathology and the irrefutable genetic 'truth' is articulated not just in technical form but in health settings that are contextualised in policy and resource by public health formulations. In turn, global health concerns of the kind I discuss in the early chapters of this book are framed by the predictive capabilities of health science, and the discursively formulated South Asian 'ethno-racial' risk package. As the racial genetic gaze (Gilroy 1998) recodifies cultural ideas into static and truth-making certainty, the scientific 'reality' of the gene occupies a curiously ambiguous position. As Lock (2007) has argued, the massive variability of gene–environment interactions means that there is a universe of possibilities inherent within the field of 'knowability'. Such precariousness in knowledge cannot possibly be welded in any certain confidence with already problematic, socially and politically constructed categories of racialised difference. And yet, as Braun (2002) indicates in echoes of many other writers, such naturalisation of racial and ethnic difference is plentiful, and functions to draw a misleadingly opaque lens over the vast, complex, and multifactorial interactions of social structures, biographies, and mechanisms of biology. As I have drawn attention to above using my own biographical identity, explicit statements about South Asians being genetically predisposed to diabetes confuse a range of ethno-linguistic, social, historical, and geo-political identities, melds them into an explanatory catchall, turning, as Montoya (2011) argues, a social label into a natural label.

Over the course of the book, I have attempted to frame the South Asian diabetes health risk not as an objectively viewed, static, and standalone scientific and public health issue, but rather as a systematically formed series of practices. One could view these practices through a discursive formation (Foucault 1972) lens, focusing on the object at the centre of the gaze being formed through the practices that derive from and generate racial-genetic discourse. Given the inherently social and political nature of the science of human groups and health, as I have shown in previous chapters, the political accomplishment and socially mediated nature of risk, especially in relation to racialised groups, becomes a part of the systematic production of South Asian 'ethno-racial' diabetes risk. Advances in genetic techno-science, biomedicine, and what could be described as new forms of surveillance (Raman and Tutton 2010) at the genetic and molecular level constitute the packages of ideas which help form the practice of producing racial meaning. The convincing power of these discourses, with their constitutive cultural, lifestyle, and genetic components, is worthy of social scientific address. This is especially the case when the terrain on which these knowledge-making practices sit are fundamentally socio-cultural and economic (Link and McKinlay 2009). In addition, since diabetes is not a single disease, but a cluster of conditions, with huge complications involved in even possibly substantiating a single, direct cause-and-effect relationship, untangling a human health condition deeply embedded within social situations (as with all human health) and attempting reductionist explanations using racial-genetics appears problematic. Empirical biomedical science and the scientific method are founded on controlling variables, so this raises the troublesome question of unravelling the 'social' from the genetic, given the infinite number of interactions possible (Happe 2013). When combined with what Montoya (2011) has identified and which I refer to in earlier chapters—namely, grouping human beings on the basis of quite arbitrary combinations of geopolitical, linguistic, ethnic, skin colour, categories—it appears to be problematic at best, and evidently, constructive of racialised health risks at a more serious impact level. Ironically, given that type 2 diabetes is known to be a disorder which is preventable and manageable, racial genetics offer some problematic fatalisms in the implications of a disease, starting at the genetic and molecular level, rendering the very lifestyle interventions proposed by established biomedicine as problematic.

I do not argue that racial-genetic diabetes discourse *necessarily* produces the kind of 'therapeutic nihilism' which McDermott (1998) refers to, whereby groups adopt some of the fatalism connected to biogenetic constructions, specifically non-curability. Nor do I argue that these processes operate in a linear, one-way fashion, resulting in 'docile bodies', which simply react to the application of knowledge and power. However, in accordance with the core concerns of this book, impacts on groups already experiencing the legacies of racialised health discourses should be the subject of questioning. As officially and professionally legitimated notions of genetic vulnerability become more widespread and integral to 'common sense' biomedical and health promotion practice, the ideas become accepted amongst subjects themselves as 'cultural scripts'. By this, I mean that genetic lines of causal argument undergo *cultural and social embedding*, so that groups and individuals themselves begin to understand and accept their conditions as genetic. A wide body of medical anthropological research shows the ways in which groups demonstrate their understanding of diabetes causality in ideas of 'blood' and 'heredity' (Smith-Morris 2006; Montoya 2011).

As with all situated accounts, there is a need to withdraw from the focused application of analytical lenses and step back towards a wider historical gaze—something I did in Chap. 2—as a way to contextualise the health, race, and ethnicity arena. This wider context, however, when considered from broader disciplinary interactions takes an important parallel direction in the form of social and medical anthropology's analysis of imperial, colonial, and neocolonial processes. These historically embedded forces have been, through a variety of conceptual and theoretical excavations, found to have multiple contemporary impacts in the form of lasting inter- and intra-generational damage at the individual, group, and national levels (Fee 2006; Ferreira and Lang 2006; Montoya 2011; Farmer 2004). Such long-standing impacts and the many multifaceted and multilayered methods in which trauma infects social, political, and cultural practices is, of course, not entirely applicable here to South Asian people in the UK who occupy a wide range of heterogeneous groups. However, I would contend that, given the history of UK 'race-thinking' and the troublesome nature attributed to 'othered' populations; this particular direction for racial-genetic causality is highly problematic. It facilitates the investment of meaning in static and fixed, essential readings of difference—race becomes mobilised in biological terms once again.

A further issue is related to who appears and who disappears within the epidemiological profiles of diabetes analyses. By this, I mean that South Asians are, as I have explained in earlier chapters, problematically categorised using highly contentious, and seemingly arbitrarily grouped, signifiers of geopolitical, ethnic, and linguistic notions of identity, in no specific or coherent manner. Nonetheless, they, we, are grouped as a specific health burden, actual or potential, who carry the possibilities of ill health through a number of re-codified racial signifiers—cultural and genetic. However, diabetes rates, experiences, and access to healthcare provision amongst 'White' people (I use the term knowingly to make a point) are markedly non-racialised, culturalised, and non-risk-subset-defined.

Conclusion

Determinist types of thinking have been said to be regaining interest as biological and genetic science technology advances rapidly (Graves 2015), leaving the conceptual, theoretical, and moral order of questioning lagging far behind. Similarly, Frank (2015) reminds us of Troy Duster's poignant warning in 2005 that there would be ever-increasing reductionist arguments and explanations for social phenomena that sociologists would be faced with (Frank 2015). Standing by and observing these rapidly advancing processes would be a failure to mount and mobilise properly engaged challenges, and indeed, a failure of sociology's central tenets (Frank 2015). Having already published, in 1990, his book titled 'Backdoor to Eugenics', Duster was preempting and characterising some of the processes that I have addressed here in this book, and certainly, in this chapter. That sociologists have already started researching and publishing on the basis of a newly emergent range of fields is surprising and concerning, especially since these are not simply sympathiser specialities; they are specific, 'socially' informed applications of genetic science (e.g. 'Socio-genomics' Conley et al. 2014; 'genetics-informed sociology' Guo et al. 2008). These are not incidental episodes in intellectual and academic endeavour, receding into the *backdrop* of bio-determinism, but, as Morning succinctly states, 'Harbingers of more to come' (2014: 1676).

As I have argued in this book, the 'risky' South Asian diabetic body has taken on a number of pathologisations—namely, cultural, lifestyle, and genetic as a variety of biosocial gazes derive racialised meanings from the application of constructed and mediated markers of difference. Critical social scientific perspectives of racialised identities *expand* and *elaborate* the possibilities of culture and social action in lived everyday lives. Ethno-racial diabetes, when utilising genetic 'truths', functions to *contract* and *simplify* the dynamic possibilities of cultural and social action. The move towards such a contraction, gene–environment friendly or otherwise, does not constitute a simple add-on to the existing intricacies of this area. Rather, it changes the relationship between cultural frameworks, lifestyle, genetics, and diabetes by mobilising the 'uncertainty–certainty' tensions I refer to above. I aim partly to re-establish what Atkinson (1984) defined as the intricate interrelationship between certainty and uncertainty—something sociologists and anthropologists rely on. The general fluidity and sociality of (and, therefore, the problem with) concepts such as 'culture' and 'ethnicity' is mitigated and temporarily solved by the emergent, legitimacy-proffering 'truths'. Such 'truths' appear in both scientific and lay discourse as irrefutable, thereby assigning the original racialised categories used for the genetic argument as fixed. As with all systems of knowledge-making practices, these materially embedded discursive formations could have real impacts at service provision as providers are bound by the 'truths regimes' cascading down and around the institutional practices of health meaning-making. Clinicians may tailor their advice according to contemporary policies and their own understandings of racial-genetic difference between biological bodies, and thus, race meaning-making takes priority over the many biographical, migration-related, social, and cultural factors that play pivotal roles in health status.

The rapidly changing nature of socio-political landscapes also affects health–race relations in the UK, since both simplistic recycling of biological/cultural racisms and complex genetic articulations of difference symbolise the enduring nature of racialised differences in the UK. The multiculturally and socio-economically diverse makeup of Britain provides very specific challenges to health science and public health, with an ever-increasing need for nuanced analysis. Such processes also lead to an increase in the complexity with which ideas and practices of 'culture' can be understood, whilst acknowledging, engaging with, and attempting to combat simultaneous processes of racialisation.

References

Aspinall, P. J. (2013). When is the use of race/ethnicity appropriate in risk assessment tools for preconceptual or antenatal genetic screening and how should it be used? *Sociology, 47*(5), 957–975.

Atkinson, P. (1984). Training for certainty. *Social Science and Medicine, 19*, 949–956.

Bhopal, R. (2013). A four-stage model explaining the higher risk of type 2 diabetes mellitus in South Asians compared with European populations. *Diabetic Medicine, 30*(1), 35–42. doi:10.1111/dme.12016.

Bloch, A., Neal, S., & Solomos, J. (2013). *Race, multiculture and social policy.* Basingstoke: Palgrave Macmillan.

Braun, L. (2002). Race, ethnicity, and health: Can genetics explain disparities? *Perspectives in Biology and Medicine, 45*(2), 159–174.

Conley, D., Fletcher, J., & Dawes, C. (2014). The emergence of socio-genomics. *Contemporary Sociology, 43*(4), 458–467.

Conrad, P., & Gabe, J. (1999). Introduction: Sociological perspectives on the new genetics: An overview. *Sociology of Health and Illness, 21*(5), 505–516.

Farmer, P. (2004). An anthropology of structural violence. *Current Anthropology, 45*(3), 305–317.

Fee, M. (2006). Racializing narratives: Obesity, diabetes and the 'aboriginal' thrifty genotype. *Social Science and Medicine, 62,* 2988–2997.

Ferreira, M., & Lang, G. (2006). *Indigenous peoples and diabetes: Community empowerment and wellness.* Durham: Carolina Academic Press.

Foucault, M. (1972). *Archaeology of knowledge.* London: Routledge.

Fox, R. C. (1957). Training for uncertainty. In R. K. Merton, G. Reader, & P. L. Kendall (Eds.), *The student-physician* (pp. 207–241). Cambridge, MA: Harvard University Press.

Fox, R. C. (1980). The evolution of medical uncertainty. *The Millbank Memorial Quarterly. Health and Society, 58*(1), 1–49.

Frank, R. (2015). Back to the future? The emergence of a Geneticised Conceptualisation of Race in Sociology. *The ANNALS of the American Academy of Political and Social Science, 661,* 51–64. doi:10.1177/0002716215590775.

Gholap, N., Davies, M., Patel, K., Sattar, N., & Khunti, K. (2011). Type 2 diabetes and cardiovascular disease in South Asians. *Primary Care Diabetes, 5,* 45–56.

Gilroy, P. (1998). Race ends here. *Ethnic and Racial Studies, 21*(5), 838–847.

Graves, J. L. (2015). Great is their sin: Biological determinism in the age of genomics. *The ANNALS of the American Academy of Political and Social Science, 661,* 24–50. doi:10.1177/0002716215586558.

Gunaratnam, Y. (2003). *Researching 'race' and ethnicity: Methods, knowledge and power.* London: Sage.

Guo, G., Yuying, T., & Tianji, C. (2008). Gene by social context interactions for number of sexual partners among White male youths: Genetics-informed sociology. *American Journal of Sociology, 114*, S36–S66.

Hall, S. (1996). Race: The floating signifier. Lecture at Goldsmiths College, University of London. Transcript available at: https://www.mediaed.org/assets/products/407/transcript_407.pdf. Accessed 20 Oct 2015.

Hall, S., & Gieben, B. (1992). *Formations of modernity*. Cambridge: Polity Press in association with Basil Blackwell and the Open University.

Happe, K. (2013). *The material gene: Gender, race and heredity after the human genome project*. New York: New York University Press.

Hartley, K. (2014). The genomic contribution to diabetes, briefing note: Diabetes, genomics and public health. PHG Foundation. http://www.phg-foundation.org/file/15592/. Accessed 2 Jul 2014.

Illich, I. (1976). *Limits to medicine*. London: Marion Boyars.

Keval, H. (2015). Risky cultures to risky genes: The racialised discursive construction of South Asian genetic diabetes risk. *New Genetics and Society*. doi: 10.1080/14636778.2015.1036155.

Knowles, C. (2007). Theorizing race and ethnicity–Contemporary paradigms and perspectives. In P. Hill-Collins & J. Solomos (Eds.), *The Sage handbook of race and ethnic studies*. London: Sage.

Link, C. L., & McKinlay, J. B. (2009). Disparities in the prevalence of diabetes: Is it race/ethnicity or socioeconomic status? Results from the Boston Area. *Ethnicity & Disease, 19*(3), 288–292.

Lock, M. (2007). Conclusion: Medical anthropology: Intimations for the future. In F. Saillant & S. Genest (Eds.), *Medical anthropology: Regional perspectives and shared concerns* (pp. 267–289). Oxford: Blackwell.

Mcdermott, R. (1998). Ethics, epidemiology and the thrifty gene: Biological determinism as a health hazard. *Social Science and Medicine, 47*(9), 1189–1195.

Montoya, M. J. (2011). *Making the Mexican diabetic: Race, science, and the genetics of inequality*. London: University of California Press.

Morning, A. (2014). And you thought we had moved beyond all that: Biological race returns to the social sciences. *Ethnic and Racial Studies, 37*(10), 1676–1685. doi:10.1080/01419870.2014.931992.

Navarro, V. (1978). *Class, struggle, the state and medicine*. London: Martin Robertson.

Neel, J. V. (1962). Diabetes mellitus: A thrifty genotype rendered detrimental by 'progress'. *American Journal of Human Genetics, 14*, 353–362

Novas, C., & Rose, R. (2000a). Genetic risk and the birth of the somatic individual. In M. Fraser & M. Greco (Eds.), *The Body-A reader* (pp. 237–241). London: Routledge.

Novas, C., & Rose, N. (2000b). Genetic risk and the birth of the somatic individual. *Economy and Society, 29*(4), 485–513.

Ossorio, P., & Duster, T. (2005). Race and genetics – Controversies in biomedical, behavioural and forensic sciences. *American Psychologist, 60*(1), 115–128.

Radakrishnan, R. (1996). *Diasporic mediations between home and location.* Minneapolis: University of Minnesota Press.

Raman, S., & Tutton, R. (2010). Life, science, and biopower. *Science, Technology and Human Values, 35*(5), 711–734.

Rose, N. (2009). Normality and pathology in a biomedical age. *Sociological Review, 57*(Suppl.), 66–83. doi:10.1111/j.1467-954X.2010.01886.x. ISSN 0038-0261.

Rose, N., & Novas, C. (2007). Biological citizenship. In A. Ong & S. J. Collier (Eds.), *Global assemblages: Technology, politics, and ethics as anthropological problems.* Oxford: Blackwell. doi:10.1002/9780470696569.ch23.

Schubert, L., Gallegos, D., Foley, W., & Harrison, C. (2012). Re-imagining the 'social' in the nutrition sciences. *Public Health Nutrition, 15*(2), 352–359. Available at: http://www.ncbi.nlm.nih.gov/pubmed/21729468. Accessed 13 Nov 2014.

Seabrook, J. A., & Avison, W. R. (2010). Genotype–environment interaction and sociology: Contributions and complexities. *Social Science and Medicine, 70*, 1277–1284.

Smith- Morris, C. (2006). *Diabetes among the Pima: Stories of survival.* Tucson: University of Arizona Press.

10

Conclusion

The aim of this book has been to situate the relationship between people's lived everyday experiences of a health condition—diabetes—against the wider, socio-political backdrop of discursive racialised constructions of risk. I aimed at exploring the ways in which a particular group of people think of diabetes, how it affects their daily lives, and the kinds of things they do to manage it. The varied, complex, and interconnected processes of race, ethnicity, and cultural identity have a symbolic and practical significance in how they were manifested in these 'cultural negotiations'. The workings of identities and multilayered complexities of the intersection with health can be gleaned from what people do and the way they talk about their experiences. When these experiences were contextualised by biographical histories, knowledge, and ethno-religious and cultural identities, the resulting negotiated orders were seen as part of a dynamic, flexible, adaptive, and agency-driven modality. In short, I attempted to contrast what people did with what constructions of them claimed they did or were capable of. The 'risky' South Asian diabetic body emerges as an ongoing result of knowledge-generating and meaning-making racialised constructions of the 'other'.

© The Editor(s) (if applicable) and The Author(s) 2016   **185**
H. Keval, *Health, Ethnicity and Diabetes*,
DOI 10.1057/978-1-137-45703-5_10

In Part 1, my aim was to provide a conceptual backdrop against which a policy and academic history of 'race-thinking' and health could be discussed. This served as a way of rerouting how we think about ethno-diabetes as a series of performative, discursive, and ideologically maintained positions. The intention of the book overall has been to ask a series of straightforward questions: How is the "problem" of South Asian health conceptualised?; How is South Asian diabetes risk framed in policy and academic discourse? What kinds of constructions prevail within these arenas? and finally What do these positions of diabetic risk look like from the perspective and experience of people within these groups? The answers to these questions are generative of alternative thinking possibilities, rather than conclusive or straightforward. In many ways, I wanted to explore what scientists have been arguably attempting to do within the frame of biomedical scientific gazes, which is address this question: How do we solve the South Asian diabetes problem? The onus on sociology and related critical social scientific enterprises is then to question this question, and excavate the layers of meaning, assumptions, and ideological nuances embedded within the framing of this (and similar) lines of query. By first, in Part 1, showing this series of constructions focused on cultural, lifestyle, and genetic arguments, and second, in Part 2, reflecting through the prism of culturally and socially negotiated practices that are counter-narratives to these constructions, it is hoped that a different way of looking at diabetes in South Asian communities emerges.

The stories and experiences people have talked about in this study were juxtaposed to the way in which health science discourse has constructed their actions, inactions, and responses to health and illness. These constructions have in the past—and in many cases, continue to—employ stereotypes of ethnicity, culture, and markers of difference. Groups characterised by heterogeneity of language, culture, and faith are often lumped together for the purposes of 'health'. The impact of this is not simply conceptual or academic—there are concrete effects on generations of people, driven by ideological and political processes. This book has aimed to highlight these constructions by identifying the main types of explanation and 'education' provided by these discursive arenas: lifestyle, genetics, and culture. By exploring people's accounts of their lives, and how diabetes sits within a bigger 'life' scheme of lived experiences, it is possible to discern how the social action demonstrated can be artic-ulated as 'resistance' to discursive, racialised constructions of passivity. Through the situated, 'culturally validated' qualitative methodology used, people's stories are seen as resistant to the dominant, discursive arenas which maintain stereotypes of 'ethnic' health. Far from being passive, the participants utilised a variety of social, cultural, ethnic, religious, and biographical resources around them—as a matter of routine and everyday occurrence. It is within these manifestations that culture, in its dynamic and flexible capability, is shown as a tool kit to manage, survive, and live in a changing landscape. The experiences, histories, biographies, and notions of identity which people had were constantly in use in the rou-tine management of diabetes.

In Part 2 of the book, a number of themes emerged: the double check-ing of the diagnosis via connections overseas using printed media and social networks (Chap. 6); the syncretic use of allopathic, traditional, and herbal remedies mediated by a historical, familial knowledge of remedies (Chap. 7); and a current and immediate engagement with the system via local, social connections and the mapping of experiences in Africa and India to experiences of migrating to this country (Chap. 8). These are all temporally mediated within biographical contexts, but utilised to deal with contemporary social landscapes. Rather than see these demonstra-tions of action as static and fixed, we can, within this study, situate them in a wider context. The use of herbs and traditional remedies (Chap. 7) comes about not simply as a taken for granted information compart-ment, but rather as a socially, culturally, historically, and temporally maintained interaction, which works with biomedicine and not against it. Sometimes, participants would use traditional medicines, combined with allopathic medicine; sometimes, they would reject the traditional because there was no objective evidence about its efficacy.

The mediation of food (Chap. 6), which is a fundamental component of diabetes management, is also something which some health discourses have a tendency to problematise, and indeed, culturally pathologise. Minority communities are often characterised as unwilling and/or unable to comply with 'health' messages and promotion. However, social actors are clearly not either compliers or non-compliers—but rather, engage in the process of social and cultural negotiations. Situations are assessed, reactions are gauged, connections to a community, family, or individuals are metered, and the action of participating is contingent upon these processes. All of these provide a counter-balance to the forms of discursive constructions of risk, which are reproduced and maintained in various guises. These elements of 'knowledges' (Ferreira and Lang 2006) and what others have called 'subjugated knowledges' (Erel 2007) form the 'resistance' and emergent counter-narratives which empower people to actively negotiate their health and illness states. Participants spoke about experiences of racism, struggle, building communities, families, but also shared interactions with people in their localities—South Asian and White, thus reflecting complex modes of multicultural interaction. They demonstrated that the things they actually did to cope with the illness were varied, numerous, and consistent with their (stable and fluid) ideas of who they were in the context of their past and the present. This was a constantly negotiated order, utilised effectively to actively assess their health and illness states—specifically, their diabetes. The observation of social actors and their dynamic roles in shifting, sometimes precarious, social landscapes, as is the case for South Asian migrants who are part of the history of British race relations, reveals complex diasporic and transnational notions of belonging. Such identity (re)formations emerge not as isolated from health and illness states, but, as Blaxter argues, 'a grid through which health and illness are perceived and given meaning' (2004: 170).

A major aim of this book was to problematise the area of race and ethnicity in health research. The idea of race and its use in policy, academic research, and political rhetoric was integral to the context I attempted to establish in Part 1. However, race is not an issue which can be resolved once and for all since, as Duster maintains incisively, there is a powerful need to examine '"ordinary" research in which race is embedded because it is unexamined, and unexamined because it is embedded' (2000: xiv). The notion of difference and similarity being embedded within the methodology of this study should not be confined to this compartment. Difference—and here, I invoke racialised categories of culture and genetics as they appear in discourse—is, as Duster tells us, embedded fully in the very fabric of health discourse.

The use of a situated, 'culturally validated' method of interacting and co-producing interactions has, I hope, contributed to the study of this endlessly accomplished socio-cultural landscape. At a methodological level, the process of 'cultural validations' characterises interconnections between various facets of identity occurring within the field. This is not a static and delimited 'box' within which difference is 'dealt' with, but points to a wider acknowledgement and embracing of the notion of cultural identity and ethnicity as proccessual contexts. They cannot be limited to encounters, but characterise whole research contexts. Investigating states of health and illness, there is always a requirement to look outside the individual and observe and locate those structures which impact upon the person's life (this is clear from early work by Blaxter 1983; Herzlich and Pierret 1987). What people were saying about their diabetes necessarily has to be placed in a social and cultural context, with specific reference also to ethnicity, life experiences, and history. For example, it represents one dimension to describe what people feel, and then, do about their diabetes, but represents a different dimension when these same people talk about how their management 'tools' were developed, where they acquired information, and what kinds of connections they still had with the countries they migrated from, as well as their personal locations in history. When we then view these articulations against the backdrop of epidemiology, biomedical science, academic and government health discourse, the two strands become linked in counter-resistance tension. In effect, participants are far from limited to the biological and cultural deficit category they are often allocated.

Discursive Constructions, Embodied Resistance

Chapters 6, 7, and 8—namely, the diagnosis, diet and food routines, the use of complementary, traditional, and herbal remedies, and the notion of cultural identity, community, and biography—help us to frame diabetes differently to the versions prevalent in many contemporary discursively constructed arenas. We need to acknowledge that, first, the experience of diabetes is far more complex in a culturally and socially situated way than is taken for granted by either solely biomedical or health intervention research. Second, using various mechanisms within their cultural and social repertoire, people actively employ cultural negotiations in health and illness, which can be seen as forms of resistance to the constructions of South Asians prevalent in health discourse. This demonstrable resistance is generated through social and body politics. In Foucauldian terms, the body being constructed through discourses and practices (Lupton 1997) is rendered docile by the specialised and professional gaze of the medical encounter and establishment. Disciplinary power exercises its authority over the body's appearance and state, by regulation and objectification, served through observation, measurement, and comparison (Lupton 1997). However, it is also through discursive practices and the production of knowledge that a type of body (a representation) may be generated and maintained. In this book, Part 1 is intended to show that when viewed from a wider critical perspective, it is possible that various forms of knowledge production and maintenance have resulted in a form of 'risky South Asian body', as shown in academic science and health policy discourse. The people in this study were employing resistance to these overarching discourses pertaining to their bodies and their lives. The bringing alive of the previously conceptualised 'docile' body, or what constructions might indicate as the passive cultural body signals not only the re-rendering of the biological–social duality, but also the relationship between categories of difference imposed by external defining structures, and notions of ethnic identity as created, maintained, and negotiated by people themselves via cultural negotiations.

Participants often talked of the problems they faced in language barriers, experiences of racism, dominance of the medical model of diabetes treatment and the availability of information (amongst others) as issues which were faced using 'local techniques and strategies of power' (Lupton 1997: 103). It is through these forms of resistance that people were activating dynamic notions of cultural and ethnic identity. In a sense they constituted culture in all its fluidity, using whatever resources they had—including their shifting identities. Hence, they were 'making culture' as much as responding to given notions of it (Lambert and Sevak 1996).

It is possible to locate the study as a possible contribution to the structure agency issue in relation to health and ethnicity, while at the same time, emphasising, as is the constant theme in this study, the notion of 'resistance' and counter-narrative production. As Williams observed, potential and fruitful explanations in the area of health may lie in the exploration of 'reflexivity and cultural resistance' (1995: 601), and offer the intellectual and empirical challenge of recognising the dialectical interconnection of 'freedom and constraint in daily life' (1995: 601). Medical anthropologists and sociologists have used situated accounts and observed how diabetes narratives tell the story of people and their diabetes as contextualised by social and political forces (Lang 2006; Omura 2006). Perhaps within this combination of medical anthropological community empowerment models (Ferreira and Lang 2006), the 'sharing stories' notion used by Greenhalgh et al. (2005), the critical role of interconnectedness of identities in the research process and the framing of discursive risk construction, it is possible to situate this study in the wider body of work as an insight into socially and culturally contextualised diabetes experiences.

The notion of 'empowerment' brought about by the use of life-history methods in the 1980s, and key to emancipatory tools in welfare practice (Chamberlayne et al. 2000), has a particular purchase within this study. As shown above, in-depth biographical work serves to locate people as historically formed, but also, as immediate and current social actors. As Erel (2007) has demonstrated in work on migrant women, biographical methods and the analysis of storytelling have the potential for transforming what Foucault (1980) would regard as subjugated knowledges. As dominant paradigms create and maintain structural positions within which actors operate, the transformative potential of life stories, as Erel (2007) articulates, is found in the way people communicate their counter-structures— resistances—to immigration control. Here, we can discern parallels to our biographically informed social action, articulated as forms of resistance to the dominant construction of South Asian diabetic risks. Biographical life stories of the Gujarati people here and the articulation of their experiences, embedded in what people do to deal with their condition, thus, run counter to and 'challenge the positions ascribed them structurally and discursively' (Erel 2007: 9.3). It is hoped that this book contributes to a realignment of some of the traditional gazes in 'ethno-diabetes' and generates alternative ways of situating cultural, ethno-religious, and social action within the appropriate dynamic contexts of the social world.

In chapter 9, I reopened what was perhaps thought to be a closed and resolved issue, but further highlighting the many risks of mobilising racial-genetic arguments in relation to South Asian diabetes. Although the genetic predisposition line of argument has a long history, I showed in this chapter that these understandings have gained recent and powerful momentum, despite often being based on precarious and ambivalent conceptualisations and scientific footing. The impacts of reverting to older biological essentialising and reductionist racial tropes are many and varied for all of society, but for subjugated, racialised, and 'othered' populations, the impact end of this continuum is considerable.

Assigning racialised identities—cultural or genetic—is not simply an imposition of *an* identity; it is the stripping away of any other possibilities of identities so that alternatives become either impossible or very difficult to conceive and act on (Fassin 2011). As Ann Morning incisively tells us, 'measuring racial difference—like virtually every other type of scientific inquiry—involves a series of judgment calls: conscious decisions that govern how we collect and analyse complex data. Racial differences do not just "jump out" unambiguously from biological data.' (2006) The lived social and cultural dynamics of people's lives, as discussed in this book, tell us that these racial ascriptions and assignations, whilst occurring persistently at one discursive and policy level, are also ably resisted through the counter-narratives and practices of people negotiating their lives, biographies, and health. The work of critical gazes is to amplify and make visible these actions and voices.

My problematisation of the accepted, apparently conventional view of 'South Asian' diabetes rests on the risks, benefits, and potential losses of doing social research across and inside categories of difference such as race, ethnicity, and culture. Becker poses a crucial question when he considers 'racism and the research question': 'how can we avoid the mistakes we aren't aware of because no-one has yet called them to public attention?' (2000: 252). In a sense, this book poses that question for South Asian diabetes. It requests from the multifaceted 'ethno-diabetes' industry and knowledge enterprise a moment in which to critically reflect on the potentially invisible and visible processes of racialisation, and to draw back from the multisited racialising gaze. This is so that we can view the many socio-political and discursive constructions of the South Asian diabetic body from a critical vantage point, and importantly, generate a much-needed counter-narrative.

References

Becker, H. S. (2000). Afterward: Racism and the research process. In F. W. Twine & J. Warren (Eds.), *Racing research researching race – Methodological dilemmas in critical race studies*. London: New York University Press.

Blaxter, M. (1983). The causes of disease: Women talking. *Social Science and Medicine, 17*, 59–69.

Blaxter, M. (2004). Life narratives, identity and health. In D. Kelleher & G. Leavy (Eds.), *Identity and health*. London: Routledge.

Chamberlayne, P., Bornat, J., & Wengraf, T. (Eds.). (2000). *The turn to biographical methods in social science*. London: Routledge.

Duster, T. (2000). Foreword. In F. W. Twine & J. Warren (Eds.), *Racing research researching race – Methodological dilemmas in critical race studies*. London: New York University Press.

Erel, U. (2007). Constructing meaningful lives: Biographical methods in research on migrant women. *Sociological Research Online, 12*(4). http://www.socresonline.org.uk/12/4/5.html

Fassin, D. (2011). Racialisation: How to do races with bodies. In F. E. Mascia-Lees (Ed.), *Companion to the anthropology of the body and embodiment* (1st ed.). London: Blackwell.

Ferreira, M., & Lang, G. (2006). *Indigenous peoples and diabetes: Community empowerment and wellness*. Durham: Carolina Academic Press.

Foucault, M. (1980) *Power/Knowledge - Selected Interviews and Other Writings 1972-1977*. (Ed) C. Gordon. Brighton: Harvester Press.

Greenhalgh, T., Collard, A., & Begum, N. (2005). Sharing stories: Complex intervention for diabetes education in minority ethnic groups who do not speak English. *British Medical Journal, 330*, 628.

Herzlich, C., & Pierret, J. (1987). *Illness and self in society*. Baltimore: Johns Hopkins University Press.

Lambert, H., & Sevak, M. (1996). Is cultural difference a useful concept? Perceptions of health and sources of ill health among Londoners of South Asian origin. In D. Kelleher & S. Hillier (Eds.), *Researching cultural differences in health*. London: Routledge.

Lang, G. C. (2006). 'In their tellings'. Ethnographic contexts and illness narratives. In M. Ferreira & G. Lang (Eds.), *Indigenous peoples and diabetes: Community empowerment and wellness*. Durham: Carolina Academic Press.

Lupton, D. (1997). Foucault and the medicalisation critique. In A. Peterson & R. Bunton (Eds.), *Foucault, health and medicine*. London: Routledge.

Morning, A. (2006). On distinction. Is race real – A web forum organised by the Social Sciences Research Council. 07 Jun 2006. Available at: http://raceand-genomics.ssrc.org/Morning/. Accessed 16 Oct 2015.

Omura, E. (2006). Mino-Miijim's 'Good food for the future'. Beyond culturally appropriate diabetes programs. In M. Ferreira & G. Lang (Eds.), *Indigenous peoples and diabetes: Community empowerment and wellness*. Durham: Carolina Academic Press.

Williams, S. J. (1995). Theorising class, health and lifestyles: Can Bourdieu help us? *Sociology of Health & Illness, 17*(5), 577–604.

Bibliography

Black, D. (1980). *Inequalities in health: Report of a working group*. London: Department of Health and Social Security/Stationery Office.

Department of Health. (2002). *National service framework for diabetes: Standards*.

Foucault, M. (1988). The political technology of individuals. In L. H. Martin, H. Gutman, & P. H. Hutton (Eds.), *Technologies of the self: A seminar with Michel Foucault*. London: Tavistock.

Jobanputra, R., & Furnham, A. F. (2005). British Gujarati Indian immigrants' and British Caucasian beliefs about health and illness. *International Journal of Social Psychiatry, 51*(4), 350–364.

Karlsen, S., & Laia, B. (2012). Understanding the influence of ethnicity on health. In G. Craig, K. Atkin, S. Chatoo, & R. Flynn (Eds.), *Understanding 'race' and ethnicity: Theory, history, policy, practice* (pp. 115–132). Bristol: Policy Press.

Karlsen, S., & Nazroo, J. Y. (2002). Agency and structure: The impact of ethnic identity and racism in the health of ethnic minority people. *Sociology of Health & Illness, 24*(1), 1–20.

Kelleher, D., & Hillier, S. (Eds.). (1996). *Researching cultural differences in health*. London: Routledge.

Kelleher, D., & Islam, S. (1994). The problem of integration: Asian people and diabetes. *Journal of the Royal Society of Medicine, 87*, 414–417.

© The Editor(s) (if applicable) and The Author(s) 2016   **195**
H. Keval, *Health, Ethnicity and Diabetes*,
DOI 10.1057/978-1-137-45703-5

Neal, S., Bennett, K., Cochrane, A., & Mohan, G. (2013). Living multiculture: Understanding the new spatial and social relations of ethnicity and multiculture in England. *Environment and Planning C: Government and Policy, 31*, 308–323. doi:10.1068/c11263r.

Parsons, T. (1951). *The social system*. Glencoe: The Free Press.

Schutz, A. (1962). *Collected papers I: The problem of social reality*. The Hague: Martinus Nijhoff.

Shaw, I., & Gould, N. (2001). *Qualitative researching in social work*. London: Sage.

Sriskantharajah, J., & Kai, J. (2007). Promoting physical activity among South Asian women with coronary heart disease and diabetes: What might help? *Family Practice, 24*, 71–76.

Turner, B. S. (2014). Religion and contemporary sociological theories. *Current Sociology Review, 62*(6), 771–788.

Index

© The Editor(s) (if applicable) and The Author(s) 2016   **197**
H. Keval, *Health, Ethnicity and Diabetes,*
DOI 10.1057/978-1-137-45703-5